A Practical Guide to COVID-19 Prevention & Control for Maritime Pilots & Seafarers

船舶驾引人员
防控新冠肺炎英语手册

中国航海学会
中国引航协会　组织编写

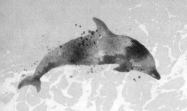

编委会

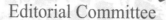

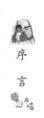

序　言

　　新冠肺炎疫情发生以来，在以习近平总书记为核心的党中央正确领导下，全国人民共同努力、众志成城，取得了国内疫情防控形势持续向好的可喜局面。但是，国内抗疫战斗尚未结束，我们既面临着疫情全球蔓延的严峻考验，也要积极复工复产，确保经济社会损失降低到最小。为此，航运领域各有关方面在确保疫情可控的条件下，努力恢复口岸正常往来，保持航运企业和船舶安全周转，加速提高船舶进出港和货物装卸效率，确保物流畅通和进出口贸易持续。

　　在这样特殊的时期，远洋船员和船舶引航人员的工作具有特殊性：他们不可避免要接触不同国家和地区的工作人员，所以加强他们的防疫知识和技能学习，提高对外沟通效率和船舶进出港效率是当务之急。"疫情就是命令，防控就是责任。"中国航海学会携手中国引航协会，发挥科技社团优势，组织国内众多一线远洋船长、高级引航员和行业专家，在《引航员防控新冠肺炎英语手册》的基础上，对内容进行扩充、改编和完善，编制完成了《船舶驾引人员防控新冠肺炎英语手册》，旨在为船舶驾驶员、引航员与外国船舶和港口相关人员交流沟通中全面做好疫情防控提供参考和便利。

　　船舶是移动的国土，海员和引航员队伍的防疫工作是全国防疫和全球公共卫生安全的重要组成部分。希望本手册能尽量满足船舶驾驶员和引航员在海上航行、靠港和执行引航任务等具体工作情境下的防控和对外高效沟通需求，为海上安全运输"生命线"保驾护航。

　　借此机会，向广大奋战在一线的抗疫医护工作者致以崇高的敬意！向全国远洋船员和引航员表示诚挚的敬意！守望相助，众志成城。祈愿春暖夏至，疫情早日结束！

中国航海学会理事长

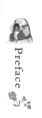

Preface

Under the correct leadership of the Central Committee of the Communist Party of China with General Secretary Xi Jinping as the core, the people of the whole nation have been working together to curb the continuing spread of the virus successfully since COVID-19 outbreak. However, the fight against the epidemic in China is not over yet. We are still facing the great challenge of its global outbreak, and need to actively resume work and production to minimize the economic and social losses as well. Therefore, all relevant parties in shipping industry strive to recover normal transportation at ports, and maintain the safe operation of shipping companies and vessels. They also work hard to enhance the efficiency of ships arriving and departing and that of cargo loading and discharging, so as to ensure smooth logistics and continuous trade at ports.

In such a special period, due to the particular

characteristics of the work of maritime pilots and seafarers, they inevitably have to contact staff from different countries or regions, so it is imperative to strengthen their knowledge and skills of epidemic prevention. It is also important to improve efficient communication and procedures of ship's entry and departure. "Fighting against the spread of the epidemic is the order, and carrying out prevention and control measures is the responsibility." China Institute of Navigation and China Maritime Pilots Association work together and organize talents such as captains, senior pilots and experts to complete A *Practical Guide to COVID-19 Prevention and Control for Maritime Pilots and Seafarers*. Based on this edition, the guide has been expanded and improved to provide prevention reference and convenience for maritime pilots and seafarers during their daily work with crew of foreign vessels and personnel from ports.

Ships are considered to be a part of a nation's territory. The epidemic prevention of pilots and seafarers is an important part of national epidemic prevention and global public health and safety. The

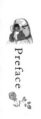

guide is designed to help pilots and seafarers to protect themselves and communicate effectively during their daily work such as navigation, berthing and unberthing, and to ensure the "lifeline" of safe maritime transportation.

I would like to take this opportunity to express my sincere gratitude and respect to medical professionals who work on the front line, as well as our hard-working pilots and seafarers all over the world. Let's help each other to fight against the epidemic. Hope the epidemic ends soon.

President of China Institute of Navigation
HE Jianzhong

编 写 说 明

新型冠状病毒引发的肺炎（COVID-19）疫情暴发以来，给中国乃至全世界带来严峻考验。中国政府高度重视疫情防控工作，全国医护人员殚精竭虑，人民群众空前团结，与疫情展开了一场艰苦卓绝的战斗。

面对突如其来的新冠病毒疫情，全国航运工作者始终坚守在海上运输最前线，不仅有序承担着我国经济贸易总量90%的货物运输，维持船舶运输和港口引航等各个重要环节的健康发展，并且秉持"外防输入、内防扩散、严防输出"的宗旨，严格做好安全防控，为保障船舶、货物、港口和人员安全作出了有效应对，也为疫情防控、民生保障和社会稳定作出了积极的贡献。

目前中国的疫情形势逐渐好转，但疫情在全球正迅速蔓延，我们既要严防国际航行船舶的输入性病例的风险，又要预防我国船员在挂靠其他港口时的被感染风险。这些迫切需要我国船舶驾驶员、引航员等从事海上运输的专业人员加强COVID-19防控知识学习，熟悉相关英语表达，以便在船舶运营和进出港口过程中与外籍工作人员有效沟通，介绍船舶疫情防控措施，交流防疫工作经验，了解疫情发展趋势，多方面共同做好防疫工作。

鉴于此，中国航海学会和中国引航协会联合组织数十位一线引航员、船长和行业专家，在《引航员防控新冠肺炎英语手册》原有内容的基础上进行了扩充和完善，在有限的时间内完成了本手册的编写工作。其中主要内容包括我国政府关于防疫工作的重要指示、国家权威部门关于COVID-19的解释和防护要求、疫情期间船舶在航或在港等情景下事关疫病防护的专业英语词汇知识等。各参编人员自愿加入、不计得失、抢抓时间、数易其稿，尤其是众多一线引航员在承担着艰巨的引航任务同时，付出了大量宝贵的休息时间，热情参与、毫无怨言、一丝不苟，携手顺利完成了编制任务。希望本手册能帮助船舶驾引人员快速掌握相关知识的常用英语表述，为我国的防疫工作贡献航运界的智慧和力量，助力我国海上"严防输出，外防输入"的重要环节，展现我国负责任的大国形象。

　　在此，特别感谢人民交通出版社杨川编辑为手册编辑排版，感谢中国人民解放军总医院李晶晶、王瑙医生参与编审工作！感谢舟山引航站引航员家属胡丹妮参与翻译编写工作。同时，我们还要衷心感谢全体业界前辈和同仁的大力扶持和鼓励。由于参编人员大多非英语专业出身，仓促之中编译难免错讹疏漏，敬请各位航海同仁谅解！如有修改意见和建议可反馈至编写人员，以便逐步修改完善，不胜感激。

编写组

2020 年 3 月 26 日

编写说明

Introduction

Since the outbreak of COVID-19, it has brought a great challenge to China and the whole world. The Chinese government has attached great importance to the prevention and control of the epidemic. Chinese people, especially medical professionals united together and made great efforts to fight against the epidemic.

Facing the sudden outbreak of COVID-19, practitioners in the shipping industry nationwide insist working at the frontline. They maintained the operation of maritime transportation orderly, which covers 90% of total amount of China's trade cargo transportation. At the same time, they took effective measures, under the principle of "preventing case imported from overseas, the spread nationwide and cases exported from China", to prevent and control the epidemic, so as to ensure the safety of ships, cargoes, ports and personnel. All these efforts have made positive contribution to the people's livelihood and social stability.

At present, China's epidemic situation gets better gradually, but the epidemic is spreading rapidly in other parts of the world. We should not only prevent strictly the risk of cases imported from international navigation ships during their stay at Chinese ports, but also prevent the risk of Chinese crew infection when their ships visit ports of other countries. It requests practitioners in shipping industry such as Chinese seafarers and pilots to strengthen the epidemic prevention and control knowledge and be familiar with relevant English expressions, so that they can communicate effectively with foreign staff, introduce and exchange relevant information, understand the trend of epidemic development, and work together to fight against COVID-19.

Therefore, China Institute of Navigation and China Maritime Pilots Association organized tens of senior pilots, captains and experts to complete this guide based on expanding and improving the first edition. The main contents include the important instructions of the Chinese government on epidemic prevention, the explanation of COVID-19 and protective requirements from national authorities, and the English terminology and expressions related to the epidemic protection for various scenarios during ships' navigation, pilotage or stay at ports. All participants voluntarily worked on this guide regardless of gain or loss. They have discussed and edited this guide for many rounds within a limited time. Especially those pilots, who need to undertake arduous pilotage tasks daily, have actively participated and done a lot work in their personal time without complaint. With great efforts of all participants, we've successfully completed this guide. The guide is designed to help pilots and seafarers master commonly used English expressions about the epidemic prevention. It is expected to contribute to the epidemic prevention from shipping community, helping to strictly prevent imported cases from and exported cases to other countries and regions and showing the responsible image of China.

We would like to express our sincere gratitude to Editor YANG Chuan from China Communications Publishing & Media Management Co, Ltd. for editing and formatting works, Doctor LI Jingjing and Doctor WANG Jin from People's Liberation Army General Hospital for helping in editing and reviewing the book, HU Danni, wife of a pilot from Zhoushan Pilot Station, for translating and proofreading. At the same time, we would like to extend our sincere gratitude to all the predecessors and colleagues for their strong support and encouragement. Any advice and criticism are warmly welcome. If there is any mistake or error, please contact us and help us to perfect this guide. Thanks a lot.

Editorial team

March 26th, 2020

目

录

目 录
CONTENTS

第4章 常用防疫语句

第 1 章 新冠肺炎简介
Chapter 1 What is COVID-19

1.1 关于新冠肺炎
About COVID-19

新冠肺炎：一种由新型冠状病毒引起的呼吸系统疾病，现在全球有多个国家发现确诊病例。该病毒被命名为"SARS-CoV-2"，其引起的疾病被命名为"新型冠状病毒肺炎"（简称为"新冠肺炎"，英文缩写为 COVID-19）。2020 年 1 月 30 日，世界卫生组织 (WHO) 宣布疫情构成国际关注的突发公共卫生事件（PHEIC），3 月 11 日，WHO 评估认为，新冠肺炎已具有"大流行病"特征。

COVID-19 (Coronavirus Disease-2019), an outbreak of respiratory illness, has now been detected in many countries. The virus has been named "SARS-CoV-2" and the disease it causes has been named "coronavirus disease 2019" (abbreviated "COVID-19"). On January 30th, 2020, the World Health Organization (WHO) declared that the outbreak of COVID-19 constitutes a Public

Health Emergency of International Concern (PHEIC), on March 11th, the WHO assessed that COVID-19 already had the characteristics of a "pandemic".

3月16日，中华人民共和国国务院联防联控机制召开新闻发布会，介绍依法防控境外疫情输入有关情况。随着WHO将新冠肺炎疫情全球的风险级别调高，中国目前亦面临有效防范境外疫情输入的挑战。交通运输部、海关总署、移民管理局及其他部门都将防范海外疫情输入风险作为当前最重要的工作，并出台一系列相关措施。

On March 16th, Joint Prevention and Control Mechanism of the State Council of China held a press conference to introduce the prevention and control of overseas epidemic disease in accordance with the law. With the WHO raising the global risk level for COVID-19 outbreak, China is also facing the challenge of preventing new cases imported from overseas effectively. The Ministry of Transport, the General Administration of Customs, the National Immigration Administration and other ministerial departments have made prevention of epidemic diseases imported from overseas the priority task at present, and have issued a series of relevant measures.

一是实施分级管理。按照国家有关部门对重点区域的判断，对船舶实施有区别的监管措施；二是开展远程非现场执法。开展对入境船舶的信息摸排，及时将我国的疫情防控政策通报给到港的船舶，同时对船舶、船员证书的状态进行远程核查，确保证书文书有效；三是加强联防联控。为海关和国家卫生健康委员会部门登船检疫、检测提供便利。同时，协调国际海事组织（IMO）、国际劳工组织（ILO）等相关的国际组织出台接受中国籍国际航行船舶展期、延期办理相关证照的政策，避免不必要的船岸人员接触。

First, classified management will be employed according to the judgment of the relevant departments of the state on key areas, and different supervision measures shall be applied to different vessels. Second, remote off-spot law enforcement will be carried out. Maritime Safety Administration（MSA）will carry out information search of incoming ships, and timely inform the incoming ships of China's epidemic prevention and control policies. Meanwhile, MSA will conduct remote verification on the status of ships and crew certificates to ensure the validity of certificates. Third, MSA will strengthen joint prevention and joint control, providing convenience for customs and health departments to board the ship for quarantine and inspection. At the same time, MSA will coordinate with the International Maritime Organization (IMO), the International Labour Organization (ILO) and other relevant international organizations to issue the policy of accepting the renewal and extension of relevant certificates and the licenses for Chinese ships of international navigation, so as to avoid unnecessary contact between the ship and the shore personnel.

1.2 新冠病毒主要传播途径和预防措施
Main transmission routes and preventive measures of COVID-19

1.2.1 主要传播途径
Main transmission routes

根据《新型冠状病毒肺炎诊疗方案（试行第七版）》:

According to *COVID-19 Diagnosis and Treatment Plan* (Provisional 7th Edition)：

（1）经呼吸道飞沫传播。患者咳嗽、打喷嚏或说话产生的呼吸道飞沫接触敏感的黏膜表面，如眼睛、鼻子或嘴时，便会发生飞沫传播。

Respiratory droplets transmission. Droplet transmission occurs when respiratory droplets generated via coughing, sneezing or talking contact susceptible mucosal surfaces, such as eyes, nose or mouth.

（2）密切接触传播。手接触有病毒飞沫沉积的物品后，再接触口腔、鼻腔、眼睛或其他黏膜组织，导致感染。

Close contact transmission. Droplets are deposited on the surface of objects. Hands can be contaminated after touching these subjects. People will be infected if they touch their mouths, noses, eyes or other mucous membranes with their contaminated hands.

（3）气溶胶传播（可能）。在相对封闭的环境中长时间暴露于高浓度气溶胶情况下，存在病毒经气溶胶传播的可能。

Aerosol transmission (possible). The virus might

spread by high-density aerosol when exposed in a relatively closed environment for a long time.

1.2.2 预防措施
Preventive measures

（1）减少或避免人际接触。

Reduce or avoid person-to-person contact.

（2）使用含酒精成分的免洗洗手液或肥皂和清水勤洗手。

Clean our hands frequently with alcohol-based sanitizer or soap and water.

（3）与咳嗽、打喷嚏的人保持安全距离。

Keep a safe distance from someone who is coughing or sneezing.

（4）佩戴必要的防护用品，如口罩、护目镜、手套等。

Wear necessary protective equipment such as face masks, goggles and gloves.

（5）保持适当通风。

Maintain proper ventilation.

（6）避免触摸口、鼻和眼等。

Avoid touching our eyes, nose, and mouth.

（7）对话时保持适当距离；如打喷嚏、咳嗽等时，要用纸巾等遮挡，事后仔细清洗手、口和鼻等。

Keep a proper distance during the conversation. Cover our mouth and nose with a tissue when coughing or sneezing, and be sure to wash our hands, mouth and nose carefully afterwards.

（8）对物品和器材进行必要的消毒，使用含酒精的消毒剂时应远离火源。

Undertake necessary sterilization for items and equipment. Keep away from fire when using alcohol-based disinfectants.

（9）如有发热、咳嗽等可疑症状，应立即隔离，并通知相关人员。

If someone have any suspicious symptoms such as fever and cough, please isolate him immediately, and then notify relevant authorities.

（10）适度锻炼，增强体质；注意休息，提高自身免疫力。

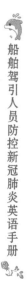

Keep doing exercises to enhance our physical status. Rest well, and try to improve our immunity.

1.3 关于新冠肺炎的重要知识点
Key points that we need to know about COVID-19

1.3.1 潜伏期
Incubation period

基于目前的流行病学调查，无症状潜伏期一般为 3 ~ 7 天，最长为 14 天。

Based on the current epidemiological investigation, the asymptomatic incubation period is generally 3-7 days, and the longest is 14 days.

1.3.2 正确洗手可减少接触传播风险
Washing hands properly can reduce the risk of contact transmission

手触摸的物品被含病毒的飞沫污染，病毒可能会经手侵入口腔、鼻腔、眼睛等的黏膜，进而增加感染风险。对物品、环境进行消毒和正确洗手都是避免传播的主要措施。

The virus may enter the mucous membranes

of mouth, nose or eyes by hand touching items contaminated by droplets, increasing the risk of infection. Main measures to avoid transmission are to disinfect items and the surroundings and wash our hands properly.

1.3.3 主要临床表现为发热、乏力和干咳
Main clinical symptoms are fever, fatigue and dry cough

少数患者伴有鼻塞、流涕、腹泻等症状。重型病例多在一周后出现呼吸困难，严重者快速发展为急性呼吸窘迫综合征、脓毒症休克、难以纠正的代谢性酸中毒和凝血功能障碍。

A few numbers of patients show symptoms such as nasal obstruction, runny nose or diarrhea. In severe cases, dyspnea usually occurs after one week. It progresses rapidly to ARDS (Acute Respiratory Distress Syndrome), septic shock, difficult-to-tackle metabolic acidosis or coagulation dysfunction.

1.3.4 少数患者没有发热症状
A few patients have no fever

值得注意的是重型、危重型患者病程中可为中低热，甚至无明显发热。危重患者虽然没有发热，但有明显的活动后呼吸急促，心慌胸闷等症状。少数患者仅表现为低热、轻微乏力等，无肺炎表现，多在一周后恢复。

It is worth noticing that severe and critical patients can have moderate to low fever in the course of disease, or even no obvious fever. But they often show other symptoms including dyspnea, palpitation or tightness in the chest. A few patients with a low fever or mild fatigue but no symptoms of pneumonia will mostly recover in one week.

1.3.5 在空气中传播距离非常有限
The distance of transmission in the air is very limited

新冠病毒在空气中传播距离非常有限，无风状态下大概 1～2 m。在干燥环境下，新冠病毒存活时间大概是 48 h。在空气中 2 h 以后，它的活性就明显地下降。

SARS-CoV-2 can be spread by air for a limited distance from 1 to 2 meters without floating in the air. It can survive about 48 hours in a dry environment.

After being in the air for 2 hours, its activity decreases remarkably.

1.4 保持手部清洁
Hand hygiene

洗手应 20 s 以上，确保洗到整个手部，如拇指、手指尖和指缝。洗手后用纸巾关水龙头。

We should wash our hands for at least 20 seconds. Make sure we have clean all parts such as our thumbs, tips of fingers and space between fingers. Use a tissue to turn off the faucet after washing our hands.

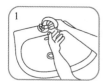

1.Wet hands with water.
淋湿双手

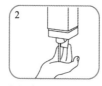

2.Apply soap to cover all of your hands surfaces.
双手涂抹适量皂液

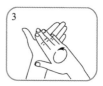

3.Rub hands palm to palm.
掌心对掌心搓擦

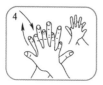

4.Rub right palm over the top of the left hand with interlaced fingers and vice versa.
掌心放在手背上，由指背向手指方向相互搓擦

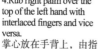

5.Rub palm to palm with fingers interlaced.
掌心相对，交错搓擦手指缝

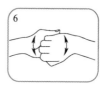

6.Rub backs of fingers to opposing palms with fingers interlocked.
两手互握，旋转搓擦

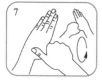

7.Continue with rotational rubbing of left thumb clasped in right palm and vice versa.
拇指在掌中旋转搓擦

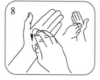

8.Continue rotational rubbing, backward and forward with clasped fingers of right hand in left palm and vice versa.
指尖在掌心旋转搓擦

9.Rinse hands with water.
用流水冲洗干净双手

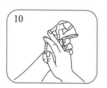

10.Dry hands thoroughly with a single use towel.
用一次性手巾擦干手

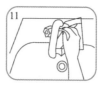

11.Use the towel to turn off the faucet.
隔着纸巾关掉水龙头

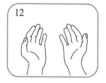

12.Now your hands are clean and safe.
这样，手就干净安全了

1.5 佩戴口罩
Wearing face masks

1.5.1 正确选择口罩
Choose the right face mask

能有效预防新冠肺炎的口罩类型有：一次性医用口罩、医用外科口罩（包括挂耳式和系带式，常见标准 YY0469—2010 或 YY0469—2011，印在口罩的独立外包装上）、医用防护口罩（如医用 GB19083—2020、KN95、 医用 N95-3M1860/1870+、FFP2-UVEX）等。

Face masks that can effectively prevent COVID-19 include disposal medical masks, medical surgical masks (ear loop and adjustable strap, frequently used standard YY0469-2010 or YY0469-2011 is printed on the package) and medical preventive masks (such as GB19083-2020, KN95, MedicalN95-3M1860/1870+, FFP2-UVEX).

1.5.2 正确佩戴口罩
Wear face mask properly

（1）日常出行建议使用医用外科口罩，如果要接触发热、咳嗽的患者建议选用医用 KN95 或 N95 口罩。

It is recommended to use medical surgical masks for daily travel, and KN95/N95 masks for contacting patients with fever or cough.

（2）佩戴口罩前应洗手，在佩戴口罩过程中避免手接触到口罩内侧面，减少口罩被污染的可能。

Wash our hands before wearing a mask, and avoid touching the inner side of the mask during wearing to reduce the possibility of contamination.

（3）注意一次性医用外科口罩有里外之分，浅色面有吸湿功能，应贴着嘴和鼻，深色面朝外，金属条（鼻夹）一端是口罩上方。

Please note that disposable surgical masks have inner and outer side respectively. The light-colored side has moisture absorption function and should be close to our mouth and nose, the dark-colored side should be outward, and the metal strip (nose clip) is at the upper part of the mask.

（4）佩戴时要将口罩折面完全展开，将嘴、鼻、下颌完全包住，然后压紧鼻夹，使其与面部完全贴合。

Please fully unfold the folded part while wearing our mask. Completely wrap our mouth, nose and jaw, and then compress the nose clip to make the mask fully fit our face.

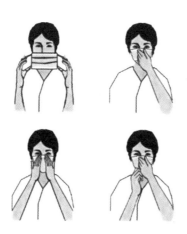

（5）口罩应定期更换，不可戴反，更不能两面轮流佩戴。

Our masks should be replaced regularly, and do not wear in reverse, not to mention on both sides in turn.

1.5.3 摘脱口罩及废弃口罩处理
Remove and dispose face mask

（1）轻轻地把口罩从脸上摘下，不要振动到口罩上的液体或固体污染物。

Remove the mask from face gently to avoid contacting liquid and solid contaminants on the mask.

（2）一只手拿住口罩系带，另一只手避免接触污染面。

Hold the mask strap with one hand and keep the other hand away from the contaminated surface.

（3）将污染面朝里折叠口罩。

Fold the contaminated surface inward.

（4）用系带将口罩系紧，之后可放入塑料袋并将袋口系紧。

Tighten face mask straps, and then place the mask in a plastic bag and fasten the bag tightly.

（5）把处理好的口罩丢入垃圾回收箱。

Throw the discarded face mask into a bin.

（6）立即清洗双手。确诊病人、疑似病人或医护工作者用过的口罩在丢弃之前要消毒。

Wash our hands immediately. Masks used by suspected patients or health practitioners should be disinfected before disposal.

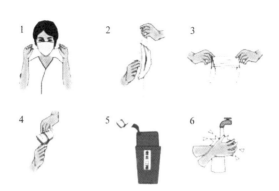

1.6 防疫问题释疑

FAQ about COVID-19

1.6.1 问：什么是冠状病毒和新型冠状病毒？

Q: What are coronaviruses and the SARS-CoV-2?

答：冠状病毒是自然界广泛存在的一大类病毒，已知会引起疾病，患者表现从普通感冒到重症肺部感染等诸多不同。新型冠状病毒是一种先前尚未在人类中发现的冠状病毒。

A: Coronaviruses are a large family of viruses that exist widely in nature, and they are known to cause diseases. Patients may suffer differently from the common cold to severe lung infection. The SARS-CoV-2 is a brand new one that has not been previously found in humans.

1.6.2 问：目前有针对新型冠状病毒的疫苗吗？

Q: Is there a vaccine against SARS-CoV-2 at the present?

答：各国正在积极的研发疫苗，有些已经开始实验，但新疫苗投入使用需要较长时间。

A: Many countries are working on the research and development of new vaccine, and some have started coronavirus vaccine testing. However, it takes a long time to produce a vaccine against COVID-19.

1.6.3 问：有针对新型冠状病毒的特效治疗方法吗？

Q: Is there any specific treatment for SARS-CoV-2?

答：对于由新型冠状病毒引起的疾病，目前没有特效的治疗方法。但是，许多症状都可以治疗，因此可以根据患者的临床状况进行治疗。此外，对感染者的支持性治疗也有积极效果。

A: There is no specific treatment for diseases caused by SARS-CoV-2. However, many symptoms can be treated, so they can be treated according to the clinical condition of the patient. In addition, some supportive treatments for the infected people are also very effective.

1.6.4 问：我要怎么做才能保护好自己？

Q: What should I do to protect myself？

答：建议保持基本的手和呼吸道卫生，以及安全的饮食习惯，尽可能避免与表现出呼吸道疾病症状(例如咳嗽或打喷嚏等) 的人密切接触。

A: It is recommended to practise basic personal hygiene and the safe eating habits. Avoid close contact with people who show respiratory symptoms such as coughing or sneezing.

1.6.5 问：人和人接触的安全距离是多少？

Q: What is the safe distance between people?

答：近距离接触时容易通过飞沫传播感染，1.5 m 到 2m 左右是比较安全的，当然距离越远越安全。

A: It is more likely to be infected through droplets during close contact, and the recommended safe distance is about 1.5 to 2 meters, which is believed that the farther the distance the safer it is.

1.6.6 问：有人可以在未发病时传播病毒吗？

Q: Can someone spread the virus without showing symptoms?

答：通常认为人们在症状最重（病得最厉害）的时候传染性最强。也有报道称：可能有一些人的传播出在有症状之前，已有报道称新型冠状病毒会发生这种情况。

A: It is generally believed that people are most contagious when their symptoms are strongest (the disease is the most severe). Reports also claimed that there may be transmission of some people before they have symptoms.

1.6.7 问：怎样判断是不是发热？

Q: How to judge whether I get a fever?

答：正常人体温一般为 36 ~ 37℃，成年人清晨安静状态下的腋窝体温 36 ~ 37℃。按体温状况，发热分为：低热 37.3 ~ 38℃、中热 38.1 ~ 39℃、高热 39.1 ~ 41℃和超高热 41℃以上。

A: The normal body temperature of human beings is generally 36-37 ℃. The axillary temperature of adults in a quiet state in the morning is 36-37℃. According to different body temperatures, there are four categories, including low fever (37.3-38 ℃), moderate fever (38.1-39 ℃), high fever (39.1-41℃), and super high fever (above 41℃).

1.6.8 问：新型冠状病毒感染的肺炎临床表现有哪些?
Q: What are the clinical manifestations of COVID-19 patients?

答：患者主要临床表现为发热、胸闷、干咳、乏力，呼吸道症状以干咳为主，并逐渐出现呼吸困难，严重者表现为急性呼吸窘迫综合征、脓毒症休克、难以纠正的代谢酸中毒和出凝血功能障碍。部分患者起病症状轻微，可无发热。多数患者为中轻症、愈后良好，少数患者病情危重，甚至死亡。

A: Main clinical manifestations of COVID-19 patient are fever, chest tightness, dry cough or fatigue. The respiratory symptoms are mainly dry cough and gradually develop into dyspnea. The severe ones have acute respiratory distress syndrome, septic shock, metabolic acidosis and hard-to-correct coagulation dysfunction. Some patients have mild onset symptoms and may have no fever. Most of patients' symptoms are mild to moderate ones and have a good prognosis. But a few may suffer from critical illnesses or even death.

1.6.9 问：目前没有出现任何不适，但是接触过疑似感染者，怎么办？

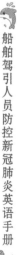
Q: At present, there is no discomfort, but I had contacted with suspected cases of COVID-19. What should I do?

答：建议居家隔离观察，观察时间为接触可疑感染者后 14 天，主要监测体温变化状况，以及观察有无胸闷、干咳、乏力等症状。

A: It is recommended to self-quarantine at home for 14 days after contacting suspected cases of COVID-19, mainly monitoring the body temperature changes and symptoms such as chest tightness, dry cough or fatigue.

1.6.10 问：近日没有出现明显发热，但出现全身酸胀或腹痛腹泻，是新型冠状病毒感染的表现吗？或者对新型冠状病毒存在易感性？

Q: I have no fever in recent days, but suffer from abdominal pain, diarrhea or soreness all over my body. Are these symptoms of the SARS-CoV-2 infection? Or am I susceptible to the SARS-CoV-2?

答：目前首发感染症状以胃肠道不适的较少，但是若出现严重的腹痛腹泻，应到医院就诊，同时注意保持营养及水、电解质的摄入平衡，此类情况下会出现机体免疫力下降，更容易受到病毒感染。

A: At present, the first symptom of infection is less likely to be gastrointestinal discomfort, but if there is serious abdominal pain and diarrhea, you should go to hospital for treatment and maintain balanced diet, appropriate water and electrolyte intake. In this case, the body immunity may decline, and you are more likely to be infected by virus.

1.6.11 问：我若出现发热、胸闷、干咳和乏力等症状怎么办？

Q: What should I do if I have symptoms such as fever, chest tightness, dry cough or fatigue?

答：最好步行（佩戴口罩，勿搭乘箱式电梯，不要采用公共交通）至最近的医疗机构进行血常规、C反应蛋白和胸部 CT 等检测，尤其是发热且伴有胸闷不适的患者，应保持高度警惕，尽早就医。

A: You'd better walk (Please wear a face mask. Don't take an elevator nor use public transportation) to the nearest medical institution for blood test, CRP and chest CT tests. Patients with fever and chest distress should stay vigilant and go to hospital as soon as possible.

1.6.12 问：如果出现早期临床表现，是不是意味着被感染了？什么情况下需要就医？

Q: If I have early clinical manifestations, does it mean that I am infected? When should I see the doctor?

答：如果出现发热(腋下体温 ≥ 37.3℃)、乏力、咳嗽、气促等急性呼吸道感染症状，或发病前 14 天内曾接触过发热伴呼吸道症状的患者，或出现小范围聚集性发病，应当到当地指定医疗机构进行排查、诊治，医生会根据发病前的活动情况、实验室检测结果等信息综合判断。因此，一旦出现疑似新型冠状病毒感染的症状，请勿恐慌，做好自身防护并及时就医。

A: If you have symptoms of acute respiratory infection such as fever (axillary temperature ≥ 37.3℃), fatigue, cough or shortness of breath,or have fever with respiratory symptoms within 14 days before you get ill, or clustered onset occurs, you should go to local designated medical institutions for screening, diagnosis and treatment. Doctors will make a comprehensive diagnosis based on the information such as your premorbid activity and laboratory test results. Therefore, once there are any suspected symptoms of coronavirus infection, do not panic and make necessary protection and see the doctor as soon as possible.

1.6.13 问：去医院就医需要注意什么？

Q: What should I do when I go to hospital?

答：就医时应如实详细讲述患病情况和就医过程，尤其是应告知医生近期的旅行和居住史、肺炎患者或疑似患者的接触史等。特别应注意的是，诊疗过程中应全程佩戴医用外科口罩或医用 KN95 口罩或医用 N95 口罩，以保护他人。

A: When you go to see a doctor, you should tell him or her how you get ill and what treatment you have done in detail. In particular, you should inform him or her your recent travel or living history, the contact history with pneumonia patients or suspected patients and so on. Special attention should be paid that you should wear a medical surgical mask or medical KN95 or N95 mask during the whole process of diagnosis and treatment, to protect others.

1.6.14 问：个人如何预防新冠肺炎？

Q: How can individuals prevent themselves against COVID-19?

答：（1）保持手部卫生。咳嗽、饭前便后、接触或处理排泄物后，要用流水洗手，或者使用含酒精成分的免洗洗手液。

A: Keep hands clean. Wash hands with running water or alcoholic hand sanitizer before a meal and after coughing, going to the bathroom, touching or handling excreta.

（2）保持室内空气流通。避免到封闭、空气不流通的公共场所和人多集中的地方，必要时佩戴口罩。

Keep our living spaces ventilated properly. Avoid going to enclosed, poor ventilated public or crowed places. Wear masks if necessary.

（3）咳嗽、打喷嚏时使用纸巾或用手肘遮掩口鼻，防止飞沫传播。

When coughing or sneezing, use a tissue or bend our elbow to cover our mouth and nose to prevent the spread of droplets.

（4）就诊或陪护时，要正确佩戴医用外科口罩或医用 N95 或医用 KN95 口罩。

If you need to go to see a doctor or accompany your family or friends to the hospital, please wear a medical surgical mask or N95 or KN95 mask correctly.

1.6.15 问：新型冠状病毒感染的症状与非典型肺炎、流感、普通感冒有什么区别？

Q: What is the differences of infection symptoms among COVID-19, SARS, influenza and common cold?

答：新型冠状病毒感染以发热、乏力、干咳为主要表现，并会出现肺炎。但值得关注的是，早期患者可能不发热，仅有畏寒和呼吸道感染症状，但CT显示有肺炎现象。新型冠状病毒感染引起的重症病例症状与非典型肺炎类似。流感的临床表现为高热、咳嗽、咽痛及肌肉疼痛等，有时也可引起肺炎，但不常见。普通感冒的症状为鼻塞、流鼻涕等，多数患者症状较轻，一般不引起肺炎症状。

A: For COVID-19, the primary manifestations are fever, dry cough, or fatigue with the diagnosis of pneumonia. However, it should be noticed that early patients may not have fever only chills and respiratory infection, but CT scan will indicate symptoms of pneumonia. Severe manifestations infection cases have similar symptoms to SARS. The clinical presentations of influenza are high fever, cough, sore throat or muscle pain. Sometimes it can also cause pneumonia, but it is not common. The symptoms of common cold are nasal congestion, running nose, etc. Most patients have mild symptoms and generally do not cause pneumonia.

1.6.16 问：如果发现有船员发热，我应该怎么做？

Q: What should I do if a crew member is found having a fever?

答：应立即对该船员采取隔离措施，并向代理和交管中心报告，等待相关工作人员和医务人员上船检查核实该船员是否感染新型冠状病毒，切不可心存侥幸。

A：The crew member must be isolated immediately. At the same time, you should report to the agent and VTS, and wait for the relevant staff and medical professionals who will board vessel and check whether the crew is infected with the virus. No one can take any chances.

第 2 章
Chapter 2

船舶疫情防控
COVID-19 Prevention and Control Onboard

2.1 船员心理波动风险防范
Risk prevention for crew's mood fluctuation

2.1.1 及时传递、宣传和解读相关部门提供的疫情信息和防控要求，普及疫情防控知识，增强自我保护能力。通过提高防范意识，早发现、早隔离、早控制，杜绝隐瞒，避免交叉感染，疫情是可防可控的。The epidemic information, prevention and control requirements provided by relevant departments should be delivered, reviewed and publicized promptly.It helps equip crew members with COVID-19 prevention and control knowledge and improve their self-protection skills. As long as we enhance our protective awareness, the outbreak can still be prevented, and contained through early detection, early quarantine, and early control.

2.1.2 做好受疫情影响无法换班船员的思想工作，取得他们对特殊时期采取特殊安排的理解，尽可能帮助他们解决生活和工作中存在的困难或问题。

Help to ease crew members when they face an extension of service period in such a challenging time. Try our best to assist them and solve their life and work difficulties or problems.

2.1.3 梳理在船船员日常居住地，重点关注来自疫情严重地区的船员，为他们了解所在地疫情发展情况提供便利，尽可能提供急需的帮助，随时关注船员的情绪变化。主管人员要对他们的工作做好兼顾和提醒，确保人身安全和船舶安全。

Have a clear picture of where crew members come from, especially those from severely affected areas. Provide convenience for them to learn about the development of the epidemic situation in their hometowns. Offer them as much help as possible and care about their emotional changes at all times. Their supervisor should balance their workload and remind them when necessary, ensuring their health and the safety of the ship.

2.1.4 船员抵港有必需品采购需求时，应提前与港口代理取得联系，请他们代为采购，解决应急所需。

If crew members need to purchase necessities in the port, they should contact their port agent in advance and ask the agent to purchase for them.

2.1.5 保障船舶内部和抵达港口（岸基提供的）Wi-Fi设备的可靠运行，确保船员有畅通渠道获得所关心的外部信息，保持信息的公开透明，不给谣言留机会，有利于缓解船员的焦虑情绪。

Keep a reliable performance of WI-FI devices on board and those provided by the shore, so that crew members can have access to external information they concern. Keep information open and transparent so that there is no room for rumors, which help the crew to relieve anxiety on board.

2.2 船员健康风险防范
Health risk prevention for crew

2.2.1 合理规范使用口罩、消毒水等防护用品。废弃的口罩，经消毒装袋后，通常按塑料垃圾处理；如果口罩使用者出现新冠肺炎确诊或疑似症状，则用过的口罩应作为医用废（弃）物，必须由岸上专门机构回收后统一处理。

Properly use face masks, disinfectants and other limited protective equipment. Used masks shall be treated as plastic waste. Once suspected cases occurred, those masks shall be treated as medical waste and only licensed company should collect, transport and do the final disposal.

2.2.2 做好船舶的公共卫生，加强公共场所的清洁和消毒工作。

Enhance the public health on board and strengthen efforts in cleaning and disinfecting in public areas.

2.2.3 注意个人卫生，及时清除垃圾，适时开窗通风，增强空气流通。外出佩戴口罩，增强自我保护意识。

Practice high standards of personal hygiene, dispose of garbage timely, and open windows for ventilation. Wear masks when going out and enhance self-protection awareness.

2.2.4 勤洗手。在咳嗽或打喷嚏后、制作食品之前、吃饭前、上厕所前后、手脏时、接触他人或外出回来后，尽快用洗手液进行规范的流水洗手。

Wash our hands frequently. According to standardized procedures, wash our hands with hand sanitizer under running water after coughing or sneezing, contacting others, returning from outside and making hands dirty, or before cooking, eating, and going to the toilet (and afterwards).

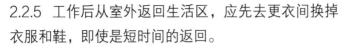

2.2.5　工作后从室外返回生活区，应先去更衣间换掉衣服和鞋，即使是短时间的返回。

Be sure to change clothes and shoes in the changing room when returning to the living area from outside, even only for a very short time.

2.2.6　在擦眼睛、嘴或鼻子以前，要确认手是干净的，眼口鼻是新冠病毒进入人体的主要突破口。

Make sure our hands are clean before wiping our eyes, mouth or nose, as they are the main gateways for viruses entering the human body.

2.2.7　勤洗热水澡。

Bath or shower frequently with warmer water.

2.2.8　所有船员要严格执行疫情期间"全体船员不得下地"的规定，这不仅是船员个人的疫情风险，更关系到集体的安危。

All crew members should follow the regulation that no one is allowed to go ashore during the epidemic outbreak. It not only relates to the individual health, but also poses a threat to all crew members ourselves.

2.2.9　保持良好的作息和饮食，避免疲劳，保持乐观的精神状态和充沛体力，这是抵抗病毒入侵的最强有力武器。

One can fight against the virus by keeping a healthy diet and sleep habits, avoiding fatigue, and maintaining good mental and physical health.

2.2.10 梳理船上药物情况，储备适量的感冒、咳嗽、发热、呕吐腹泻和抗病毒药物。新冠肺炎暂时没有特效药，根据症状服用相关药物进行临时的控制是有必要的。

Make a detailed inventory check on medicines on board. Prepare an appropriate stock of medicines for cold, cough, fever, vomiting, diarrhea and some antiviral drugs. There is no magic pill for COVID-19 and it is necessary to take temporary treatment according to the symptoms.

2.3 引航员登离船的风险防范
Risk prevention for pilots on and off board

2.3.1 负责接送引航员的船员应全程佩戴口罩，在引航员攀登邻近入口时适当后退，为引航员大口喘气或佩戴口罩留出所需空间。

Officers or crew members responsible for assisting

pilot embarkation and disembarkation should wear face masks throughout the whole process, and step back to leave enough space in case pilots need to breathe in short pants and/or put on face masks before climbing on board.

2.3.2 引航员经测量体温正常，方可前往驾驶台。

Pilots should be led to bridge if their body temperature is normal.

2.3.3 接送过程中，建议放慢步行和爬楼梯的步伐，避免因呼吸急促而揭开口罩大口呼吸。

During the transfer process, it is recommended for pilots and crew to slow down the pace of walking and climbing up the ladder to avoid taking off their face masks for air because of shortness of breath.

2.3.4 应避免引航员进入船员生活区，从舱外楼梯绕道进入或离开驾驶台。

Pilots should enter or leave the bridge via stairs outside the accommodation area and avoid entering the accommodation area.

2.3.5 船员与引航员共事期间应佩戴口罩；驾驶台保持通风；人员间保持合适的距离，处于下风时间隔应

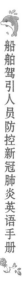

更大，并迎风左右错开。

The bridge team should wear face masks while working with pilots. Keep windows and doors open on bridge for ventilation. Remain an appropriate distance from each other. When you stay on the lee side, please widen the distance and stand relatively on left or right side.

2.4 航行安全特别注意事项
Key precautions for safe navigation

2.4.1 驾驶台团队应注意佩戴口罩后有声音变小不利收听的影响，适当提高音量发布命令、重复命令和回复命令，集中精力倾听，命令存疑时要提醒并核实。

The bridge team should be aware that wearing a face mask may muffle your voice, so please speak louder when giving, repeating and replying instructions, listen carefully and remind each other to confirm the instructions.

2.4.2 长时间佩戴口罩会导致疲劳，可轮流到室外空旷处摘口罩深呼吸调节。

Wearing face masks for a long time may cause fatigue, please take turns to remove our face mask and take a deep breath in an open outdoor space.

2.4.3 注意佩戴口罩对眼镜和使用望远镜的影响，使用时屏住呼气可降低对眼镜和望远镜的影响。戴护目镜也会起雾，影响视觉瞭望，建议使用防雾护目镜。

Wearing a face mask can impact the effectiveness of glasses and binoculars, but we can try to hold our breath to avoid blur effect temperately. Similarly, wearing a safety goggles may face the same problem and cause a blurry vision, so it is recommended to use anti-fog goggles instead.

2.5 外来人员进入的风险防范
Risk prevention for visitors' entry

2.5.1 值班人员要佩戴口罩，按《国际船舶和港口设施保安规则》(ISPS)要求严格控制外来人员，不握手，保持安全的距离，对不佩戴口罩的上船人员进行劝离。

Crew on duty should wear face masks and strictly control external access in compliance with *the International Ship and Port Facility Security Code* (*ISPS*) requirements. No hand shaking with visitors but keep a reasonable distance. Crew on duty should persuade those who do not wear face masks to leave.

2.5.2 靠泊后，生活区保留一个进出通道，其他通道全部封闭，并指定外来人员专用卫生间；对该通道和专用卫生间进行高频次的清洁和消毒（视外来人员进出情况确定频次）。

After berthing, only one passageway should be kept open to the accommodation area while the others are all closed. An exclusive toilet is reserved for visitors in the accommodation area. Depending on the visiting frequency, both the passageway and the visitors' toilet should be cleaned and disinfected regularly.

2.5.3 除非梯口值班人员能同时兼顾梯口值班和进入生活区通道控制，否则应安排专人对生活区进出通道进行 24 小时值守。

A crew member should be assigned to watch the entrance to the accommodation area around the clock, unless the one on duty at the gangway can handle it at the same time.

2.5.4 接待港口官员或业务人员来船时，可在离入口通道最近处临时摆放桌椅，作为接待场所。避免外来人员乘坐电梯。

A temporary reception desk near the entrance can be used during the visit of port officials and service providers. No lift is permitted for visitors.

2.5.5　除非必须，送物料、备件、伙食的人员不得进入生活区；避免在有疫情港口进行修理、检验和供应；必需的修理、检验和供应人员，应选捷径进入，如驾驶台的修理，从舱外楼梯进入，从而避免进入生活区。

Spare parts and provision suppliers should not enter the accommodation areas unless necessary. Reparation, inspection and supplies should be avoided at coronavirus-stricken ports. Repairers, inspectors and suppliers should go straight to their working sites for necessary work only. For bridge repairs, technicians should enter or leave the bridge from the outdoor stairway and avoid entering the accommodation area.

2.5.6　对于代理等岸基服务人员，尽量减少面对面的近距离交流，如有可能，详细的交流可以通过电话或其他方式进行。

Please minimize face-to-face engagements with shore-based service providers such as agents. Alternatively, you can communicate over the phone or by other devices if necessary.

2.6 船员室外工作的风险防范
Risk prevention for crew working outdoors

2.6.1 在靠泊期间需要在室外工作的船员,应佩戴口罩。
Crew members who need to work outdoors should wear face masks during the port stay.

2.6.2 与外来人员保持足够的距离,一般 1.5 米以外。
Keep a sufficient distance away from visitors, generally over 1.5 meters.

2.6.3 一旦发现外来人员工作过程中取下口罩的,要作提醒,必要时通过合理途径反映情况,并保持远离,尤其要避免处于他的下风侧。
Remind visitors to put on their face masks properly if they take them off during work. Report the situation in a reasonable way when necessary, and stay away especially when standing at his lee side.

2.7 离港后注意事项
Precautions after departure

2.7.1 及时与下一港代理保持联系,知悉港口在防控疫情方面的要求，如遇到可能影响船舶运行的特殊要求时，应迅速报告船舶管理公司，获取岸基支持或进一步指示。

Keep in close contact with the agent of next port of call to learn about the port's requirements for the epidemic prevention. If there are some particular requirements that impact ship operation and schedule, please report to the shipping management company for shore-based supports or further instructions.

2.7.2 配备和使用伙食、淡水时要留有余地，对疫情可能带来的不确定性要有预期，做好应有的战略储备。

A necessary strategic reserve of provisions and fresh water should be made, preparing for the potential supply shortage associated with the outbreak.

2.7.3 离开码头以后，立即组织船员和对涉外区间进行清洁消毒，对工作服、手套、安全帽等和防护用品进行消毒清洗。

After leaving the terminal, organize crew members to clean and disinfect the spaces that have been visited by others immediately. Wash and sanitize protective equipment such as workwear, gloves and safety helmets.

2.7.4 保持每日监测船员体温，做好记录并签字保存；对在港期间船舶疫情防范措施的落实情况拍照留存。船员的上船日期记录，可以成为船舶落实疫情控制的证据，也可以为船舶抵达后续港口可能面临的各类检查做好充分准备。抵港后以不怠慢、不逃避和不隐瞒的负责任态度，配合港方的防控工作。

The body temperature of all crew members should be checked and recorded every day. Photos of prevention against COVID-19 during our stay in the port should be filed. Records including the boarding log of crew members can be powerful evidence to show our efforts on COVID-19 prevention and control on board, and offer convenience for all kinds of inspections at the future ports of call. Cooperate with port authorities on the prevention and control responsibly.

2.7.5 未雨绸缪，提前准备好隔离病房。选一间生活设施和通信设施完善，能切断公共通风系统，对周边船员影响较小的房间作为隔离病房。

Precautions should be taken such as a quarantine ward. Please choose a cabin that is best suitable for isolation. It should be well-equipped with living and communication devices and an independent ventilation system in an attempt to minimize the impact on the surrounding crew members.

引航疫情防控
COVID-19 Prevention and Control During Pilotage

3.1 中国引航协会疫情防控指导措施
China Maritime Pilots Association's Guide on COVID-19 Prevention and Control

　　由于被引船疫情的不确定性、引航工作的不可替代性和不能避免接触的特殊性，做好引航职工防控新冠肺炎疫情的工作刻不容缓。为指导各引航机构做好疫情防控工作，保护引航员的生命安全和身体健康，降低被引船输入性新冠肺炎风险，有力保障水路货物运输和维护正常港航生产秩序，中国引航协会制定了《关于防控被引船输入性新冠肺炎风险的应对措施》。

　　Due to the risk of infection on board, the irreplaceability of pilot jobs and the inevitability of physical contact during work, it is urgent to enhance the prevention and control measures. China Maritime Pilots Association issued *The Prevention and Control Measures for Imported COVID-19 Infections from Ships under Pilotage* in order to guide pilot stations to prevent and control COVID-19, protect pilots' safety and health, reduce the risk of cases imported from ships, guarantee waterway transportation and maintain normal operation at local ports.

3.1.1 实施船舶分类管理
Implementation of classified management

按照全球新冠肺炎疫情发展程度以及船员的健康状况，对来自不同国家和地区的船舶实行分类，以制定相应防控措施和引航计划。

Ships from different countries or regions are classified according to the global evolution of COVID-19 and health conditions of crew members onboard so as to develop corresponding measures and pilotage plans.

（1）第一类。被引船船员有发热、咳嗽等呼吸道感染症状的疫情或疑似疫情；如该船员来自确诊人数和现存新冠肺炎病例较多的国家和地区（以下简称疫情高发国家和地区），应更加引起重视。

The first category. If any crew member has respiratory infection symptoms such as fever or cough, especially when he came from high-risk countries or regions, more attention should be paid.

（2）第二类。被引船14天内挂靠过疫情高发国家或地区的港口；船上有来自疫情高发国家和地区的船员在14天内上船工作；有船员在14天内从疫情高发国家和地区港口登船工作。

The second category. If the vessel being piloted has visited high-risk countries or regions within 14 days, or if there are crew members coming from high-risk countries or regions within 14 days, or if there are crew members boarding at ports of high-risk countries or regions within 14 days.

（3）第三类。除上述两类船舶以外的被引船。

The third category. Vessels other than the above two categories.

3.1.2 引航机构
Pilot stations

引航机构要积极开展疫情防控工作，配合海事和海关检疫部门的工作，全面加强疫情防控。

Pilot stations should carry out the prevention and control measures of the epidemic actively, cooperate with the MSA, the Quarantine departments, and comprehensively strengthen the prevention and control work.

（1）详细掌握核实被引船和船员的信息。

Get reliable information about the vessel and her crew members.

（2）建立"防疫工作日志"，对疫情排查和日常防控工作进行记录。

Establish Epidemic Prevention Log to record the epidemic investigation and the routine prevention and control measures.

（3）利用网络等多种方式，减少不必要的引航职工聚集。

Reduce unnecessary pilots gathering by online applications and resources.

（4）保证防疫物资储备和供应。

Ensure the reserve and supply of epidemic prevention equipment and materials.

（5）监测有疑似症状的引航职工。

Monitor pilots who may have suspected symptoms.

（6）做好公共场所、引航员接送车船的消毒工作，并做好记录。

Disinfect public areas, transportation cars and/or

boats, and keep records.

3.1.3 引航员
Pilots

（1）引航员应自带饮用水和食品，并区别对待三类被引船。引领第一类被引船时，穿戴防护服、护目镜、高级别医用口罩（单位自定）、手套等；引领第二类被引船时，佩戴护目镜、高级别医用口罩（单位自定）、手套，建议穿防护服；引领第三类被引船时，佩戴普通医用口罩、手套等。

The pilot should bring his own drinking water and food and treat the three categories of ships differently. When piloting the first category of ships, he should wear protective clothing, goggles, a N95 or KN95 face mask or surgical mask and latex gloves. When piloting the second category of ships, he should wear goggles, a N95 or KN95 face mask and surgical gloves. It is recommended to wear protective clothing, disposable waterproof shoe covers and disposable headwear. When piloting the third category of ships, he should wear surgical masks, gloves, etc.

（2）登船后，根据气象及船舶实际情况，尽可

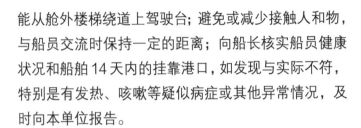

能从舱外楼梯绕道上驾驶台；避免或减少接触人和物，与船员交流时保持一定的距离；向船长核实船员健康状况和船舶 14 天内的挂靠港口，如发现与实际不符，特别是有发热、咳嗽等疑似病症或其他异常情况，及时向本单位报告。

If possible (based on the weather and the actual condition of the ship), try to take the outside stairs to the bridge after boarding, and to avoid entering the accommodation area, reduce or avoid physical contact with people or objects and keep a proper distance with crew members during face-to-face communication, verify the health conditions of the crew and the ports of call in the last 14 days with the master, and report to the pilot station in time if any inconsistency has been found, especially suspected symptoms such as fever, cough or other abnormal conditions.

（3）引航工作时，如有可能，引航员可向船长提出，引航员与船员使用不同的雷达、ECDIS、VHF和其他设备等。要注意戴口罩防疫对引航工作的影响。

When piloting, if possible, the pilot may suggest the master not to use the same radar, ECDIS, VHF and other equipment. Be aware of the influence of wearing a face mask during work.

（4）引航结束离船后，使用过的防疫物品应妥善处理，应对引航装备进行必要的消毒。如获知被引船船员有确诊或疑似新冠肺炎的病例，应自觉和配合单位进行相应的隔离。

Upon completion of a pilotage, all protective items used should be disposed properly. Pilot equipment should be disinfected. If any crew member is confirmed or suspected case of COVID-19, the pilot should be quarantined according to the requirement of local pilot station.

（5）发现自己或家属有发热、咳嗽等症状，密切接触者确诊或疑似新冠肺炎，均应及时向本单位报告；绝不带病引航，避免交叉感染。

If you and your family members have fever, cough or other symptoms, or if you have contacted any confirmed or suspected case of COVID-19, you should report it to your office immediately, and avoid working with illness and infecting others.

（6）应避免到封闭、空气不流通或人群密集的公众场所活动；咳嗽、打喷嚏时使用纸巾或用手肘遮掩口鼻，防止飞沫传播；减少人员直接接触，降低交叉感染的可能性。

Avoid entering any closed, poorly ventilated or crowded public place. Use a tissue or bend our elbow to cover our mouth and nose when coughing or sneezing to prevent droplets transmission. Reduce close contact and the possibility of cross-infection.

（7）应配合港区、海关检疫部门、船方等对疫情防控监测的工作，包括填写健康申明卡等。

Pilots should cooperate with port authorities, Quarantines and ships in monitoring prevention and control of the epidemic, such as filling in the Health Declaration Form.

3.2 引航机构疫情防控
Epidemic prevention and control at pilot stations

3.2.1 由于工作环境的特殊性，引航员每天都要面对来自不同国家和地区的船员，本着对引航员、船员身体的安全以及船舶、港口安全负责的态度，对引航员实行严格的防护措施尤为重要。

Due to the special working environment, pilots need to meet people from various countries or regions. For the safety of pilots, crew members, as well as ships and ports, it is particularly important to implement strict protective measures for pilots.

3.2.2 调整或取消引航员轮休计划，避免或减少人员流动。

Rearrange or cancel the pilot rotation plan to avoid or reduce the staff movement.

3.2.3 引航员待班期间，不坐班、不聚集，分开就餐。

During standby time, pilots are requested not to stay or gather in the office and they should have their meals separately as well.

3.2.4 监测引航员身体状况，包括有无发烧、咳嗽等疑似症状，若有疑似症状立即隔离并通知相关部门。

Monitor pilots' health conditions including whether they have a fever, cough or other suspected symptoms. If there exists any suspected symptom, isolate him and notify the relevant departments immediately.

3.2.5 严格体温检测。每次引航员坐上接送车辆之前，司机都要对引航员进行体温检测，并记入日志；每次引航员坐上引航艇/拖船之前，船员也会对引航员进

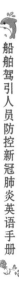

行体温检测，并记入日志。只有完成所有步骤，才允许引航员登船。

Strictly monitor body temperature. Before taking transportation vehicle, pilots should have their temperature measured and recorded by the duty driver. Same measures should be taken by the boat crew before getting in a pilot boat. Pilots cannot embark a foreign vessel until they complete all the procedures.

3.2.6 接到引航申请时，由船舶代理落实船舶和船员的信息，如是否有人员发热、有无挂靠过重点疫情港口等，经站里防控领导小组会同相关部门制定好预案后才能安排引航。

Upon receiving a pilotage application, the following information shall be confirmed with the ship's agent: Whether any crew onboard has a fever, or whether the ship has called at any coronavirus epicenter. Pilots can board the ship only after the pilot prevention and control group and relevant departments have set out a pilotage plan.

3.2.7 每日对引航员办公、居住等处所进行消毒和通风。
Disinfect and ventilate pilots' office and residence everyday.

3.2.8 注意劳逸结合，避免过度疲劳，工作中感觉疲劳或身体状况不佳时应及时报告，确保始终以良好的身体状况应对疫情，保障引航安全。

Pilots should strike a balance between work and rest, and avoid overwork. If you feel tired or uncomfortable, you should make a report immediately. Working under a healthy condition is the guarantee for safe pilotage.

3.2.9　引航结束后，根据情况或按要求安排专用车辆送至定点隔离场所休息待命。引航员隔离居住期间要勤测体温，隔离场所要勤消毒；发现身体异常应及时报告；非经批准不得擅自离开隔离居住场所。

When a pilotage is finished, pilots should be sent to a designated quarantine place by a designated car if necessary. Pilots should have their body temperature measured and living space disinfected frequently. They are requested to report any physical abnormalities immediately during the quarantine period. They cannot leave the quarantine place without permission.

3.3　引航员疫情防控
COVID-19 prevention and control for pilots

3.3.1　定时检测体温，尤其上船前。如果出现发热、咳嗽等症状应该立即报告单位和社区，并到最近定点医院发热门诊就医。

Check your body temperature regularly, especially before boarding.Symptoms such as fever or coughing should be reported to the pilot station and the community immediately. The pilot should go to the fever clinic in the nearest designated hospital for treatment.

3.3.2 引航员接到任务后，测量体温，保证身体健康；备好口罩、护目镜、手套、便携喷雾式消毒剂等防护用品。

After receiving a pilotage task, pilots should check their body temperature to ensure they are in good health condition. They should prepare protective items such as face masks, goggles, protective gloves and portable spray disinfectants, etc.

3.3.3 上船前应该佩戴好口罩、手套、护目镜等防护用品。

Before boarding, pilots should wear protective equipment such as a mask, gloves and safety goggles.

3.3.4 引领一类、二类船舶的引航员应穿戴相应的防护用品。引航结束，如需配合，待海关完成检疫并确认安全后，引航员方可离船。如果发现船员有发热、咳嗽等疑似症状，应用专车、专船艇将引航员送到指定处所隔离休息，待该船员确认没有感染，方可解除隔离。

Pilots who work on the first and the second category of ships should wear relevant protective equipment. Upon the completion of pilotage, pilots cannot leave the ship until the quarantine inspection is completed. If any crew members show symptoms of infection such as fever or cough, the pilot shall be sent to a designated place for quarantine by a designated car and/or a boat. He is free only if the crew member is confirmed of not being infected.

3.3.5 引航员执行引航任务时，必须全程佩戴口罩和手套，登离船前后应做好消毒工作；原则上一律从船舶的舱外楼梯上下驾驶台，如只能通过内通道进出，避免使用船上电梯。

Pilots must wear a face mask and gloves during pilotage. Disinfection must be done before embarkation and after disembarkation. In principle, pilots should take the detour from the stairway outside. If impossible, you can get through by the stairway inside, and try to avoid using the elevator.

3.3.6 引航员不使用船上的杯子喝水；咳嗽、打喷嚏

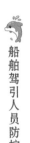

时到驾驶台外；避免与船长和船员握手等近距离接触。
Pilots should not drink with cups offered by ships during pilotage. When coughing or sneezing, pilots should go outside the bridge. They should avoid close contact such as shaking hands with the captain and crew members.

3.3.7 保持驾驶台良好通风，减少或避免接触船员和驾驶台设备。
Keep the bridge well ventilated. Reduce or avoid contacting with crew members or touching equipment in the bridge.

3.3.8 洗手要仔细，用洗手液，在流水下洗手至少20秒。
Wash your hands with soap and running water carefully for at least 20 seconds.

3.3.9 引航员登船后，应适时用75%酒精消毒，消毒时注意防火。
Pilots should use 75% alcohol for disinfection on board and beware of the risk of fire.

3.3.10 引航员应尽量避免在船餐饮及驻船，特殊情况下如无法避免需特别注意以下防护事项。

Whenever possible, pilots should avoid having meals and living onboard. Special attention should be paid to the following if it is unavoidable under special circumstances.

（1）避免在船员餐厅、驾驶台等人员密集的地方用餐，最好在引航员房间等单独空间。如航行需要必须在驾驶台，进餐时则应与其他驾驶台人员保持足够的距离（1.5 m 以上）。

You'd better enjoy your meals alone in a separate room such as the pilot cabin instead of being in crowded places such as the dining room or the bridge. When it is necessary to eat on the bridge during navigation, pilots should keep a sufficient distance of at least 1.5 meters from others.

（2）不吃生食。

Do not eat raw food.

（3）引航员应自带水杯。有条件的，可以使用一次性餐具。如不具备这样的条件，则应与船长融洽沟通，确认餐具、水杯消毒干净后方可使用，使用后再彻底消毒。

If conditions allowed, pilots should use disposable dishware and their own cups. Otherwise, they can communicate with the captain and confirm whether the tableware has been disinfected. After pilots finish their meal, all tableware should be thoroughly disinfected.

（4）运送食物和餐具人员应做好防护工作。

People in charge of meals and tableware delivery should take protective measures properly.

（5）引航员在用完洗手间后，要格外注意手部卫生。

Pilots should wash their hands thoroughly, especially after using the toilet.

（6）引航员房间使用之前彻底消毒，保持适当通风。

Thoroughly disinfect the pilot room before using and maintain proper ventilation.

（7）马桶使用前后要消毒，并冲水一次。

The toilet should be disinfected before and after use, and should be flushed every time.

（8）尽量不去其他与工作无关的场所。

If possible, pilots should stay away from other non-work related places on board.

第 4 章
Chapter 4

常用防疫语句
Commonly Used Sentences about Prevention for COVID-19

4.1 驾引人员常用语句

Common sentences for pilots and seafarers

4.1.1 早上好，船长，欢迎来到本港口。

Good morning, Mr. Captain. Welcome to our port.

4.1.2 疫情时期，请原谅我不能与你握手。

Please excuse me for not shaking hands with you in such pandemic circumstances.

4.1.3 我们保持 1.5m 以上的距离说话，如果没有听清楚，请告诉我。

Please keep social distance for at least 1.5 meters while talking, please let me know if you cannot hear me clearly.

4.1.4 船长，如果你不介意，请把驾驶台侧门打开以便通风，请关掉驾驶台的中央空调出风口。

Mr. Captain, would you mind opening the side door of

the bridge for ventilation and turning off the central air conditioner on the bridge?

4.1.5 船长，我们引航员在进港区前／登船前已经检测过体温，身体状况健康良好。佩戴口罩和手套仅仅是为安全需要，这只是防疫的一般要求。

Mr. Captain, we have our body temperature checked before entering the port area/boarding and we are in good health condition. Wearing a face mask and a pair of gloves is just for the safety, which is a normal requirement for epidemic prevention.

4.1.6 请你理解我佩戴口罩和手套的必要性，在保护自己的同时，也是为了保护你和其他船员的健康安全，避免交叉感染。建议船员也像我一样，佩戴有效的防护用品。

Please understand that it is necessary for me to wear a face mask and gloves. It is not only to protect myself, but also to protect you and your crews. In doing so, we can avoid the risk of cross infection, so I suggest that crew members should wear protective equipment like me.

4.1.7 请你理解和支持我们引航员在疫情时期的特殊做法。

Please understand and support the special practices of our pilots during the period of the epidemic.

4.1.8 引航员，我们一定会尽全力配合你们。

Mr. Pilot, we will try our best to cooperate with you.

4.1.9 咳嗽或打喷嚏时，请用纸巾或者肘部捂住口鼻。

When coughing or sneezing, cover our mouth and nose with a flexed elbow or use a tissue.

4.1.10 避免感染风险，守护大众健康，敬请佩戴口罩。

In order to prevent infection and keep everyone safe, please wear a mask.

4.1.11 船长，你们所戴的口罩是不能防止病毒传播的，请通知船公司或代理为你船配备防病毒外科口罩。

Mr. Captain, the face mask you wear can't effectively prevent virus transmission, Please ask your company or agent to provide anti-virus surgical masks for you.

4.1.12 船长早上好，请问你船最近有无人员出现发热、干咳、乏力、呼吸困难等不适症状？

Good morning, Mr. Captain! Do you have any crew member on board who has recently developed fever, dry cough, fatigue, dyspnea or the like?

4.1.13 我船上没有人出现发热、咳嗽症状。

No one on board has a fever or cough.

4.1.14 我是健康的，很高兴全体船员也没有发热、咳嗽等症状。

I am healthy and glad that none of your crew has any suspected symptoms such as fever or cough.

4.1.15 你船每天对全体船员做体温检测并记录吗？

Do you check body temperature for all crew members and record them every day?

4.1.16 最近 14 天里是否有船员换班？

Has any crew been changed in the past 14 days?

4.1.17 更换的新船员有来自疫情高发的国家或者地区吗？

Are the new crew from the epicenter countries or regions?

4.1.18 请问你船在之前 14 天停靠的港口有无船员下地？

Would you please tell me if any crew went ashore at last ports of call within 14 days?

4.1.19 请问船员下船是否佩戴口罩？

Did crew members wear face masks when they went ashore?

4.1.20 在之前的靠港期间，有没有外来人员出现发热或者咳嗽的情况？

During stay in previous ports, did any visitor have a fever or cough?

4.1.21 船员对预防新冠肺炎的措施熟悉吗？

Are your crew members familiar with preventive measures against COVID-19?

4.1.22 请定期给船舶驾驶台、生活区等公共区域消毒。

Please disinfect the bridge, the accommodation area and other public areas regularly.

4.1.23 建议你对生活区、人员通道、驾驶台和机舱等工作区及人员频繁接触的设备进行有效消毒，避免病毒通过接触进行传播。

It is recommended that you should disinfect the accommodation area, passages, bridge and engine room, and those frequently used equipment effectively to prevent virus spreading through contact.

4.1.24 船长引航员和码头方面已经采取了严格的防疫措施，我希望船上人员也同样认真对待。

Mr. Captain, pilots and staff ashore have implemented strict quarantine measures, and I hope you can take it seriously too.

4.1.25 你船在 A 国靠港期间与陆地人员有过接触吗？

Did any crew contact with visitors during the port stay in A?

4.1.26 A 国现在疫情较重，在那是否有船员下地？

There is a severe epidemic situation in A. Has any crew ever been ashore there?

4.1.27 由于你船来自疫情高发的国家，所以在船舶靠港之后会有检疫官员登船检查，在通过检疫之前所有人员不准下地，岸上所有的人员禁止登船，包括码头装卸工人。

Since your ship comes from the epicenter country, the quarantine officers will come on board to carry out inspection after alongside. Until the granting of the free pratique, nobody is allowed to go ashore, and no shore staff including stevedores are permitted to board this vessel.

4.1.28　由于你船有人员发热，所以我们需要先去锚地抛锚，等待检疫官员上船检疫。

Since some crew members have a fever on board, your ship is required to proceed to the anchorage and wait for the quarantine inspection.

4.1.29　具体的靠港计划和检疫计划你需要同下一个交接的引航员或者代理核实，并且靠好码头之后船舶将要接受检疫检查，请你通知全体船员提前做好准备。

For the specific berthing and quarantine plan, you need to check with the next pilot or your agent. Besides, your ship will be subjected to a quarantine check after alongside, so please inform your crew to be ready in advance.

4.1.30　船长，代理已经通知检疫部门，医生和救护车在码头等候，我会和他们保持联系。

Mr. Captain, your agent has informed the quarantine department. An ambulance with paramedics will wait at the terminal. And I will keep in contact with them.

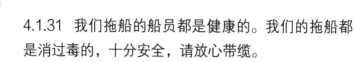

4.1.31　我们拖船的船员都是健康的。我们的拖船都是消过毒的，十分安全，请放心带缆。

All of our tug's crew members are healthy. We have sterilized all of our tug boats, and they are safe and clean. Please make fast the tug's line as usual.

4.1.32　为了你的健康，请在靠码头期间时刻保持良好的通风，尤其是驾驶台和餐厅。

For your health, please keep a good ventilation at all times during your port stay, especially in the bridge and dining room.

4.1.33　建议你靠泊后 / 离泊前做好驾驶台、通道和船员个人住所等公共场所的消毒工作，尤其要对驾驶台 VHF 和导助航设备进行重点消毒。

It is suggested that you should disinfect public places such as the bridge, passage, and crews' accommodation area after berthing or before unberthing. Especially, please focus on the disinfection of the VHF and navigational devices on the bridge.

4.1.34　靠港期间如有船员需要下地，建议不要乘坐公共交通，不要去人员密集的场所，事情办完之后尽快回船。

If any crew member need to go ashore during the port stay, it is recommended that he should neither take the public transport nor go to crowded places, and return to the ship as soon as possible after all his business has been done.

4.1.35 离港后，为安全起见，请关注你的船员体温至少 14 天。

For your safety, please monitor your crews' body temperatures for at least 14 days after departure.

4.1.36 引航员，请问这个港口 / 城市目前的新冠肺炎疫情情况如何？

Mr. Pilot, how is the epidemic situationin this port/city?

4.1.37 我们城市还无人感染。

No one has been infected in our city yet.

4.1.38 你们引航站是怎么应对这次疫情的？有什么相应的措施？对引航员有什么影响？

How did your pilot station respond to this epidemic? What are the corresponding measures? Any impact on pilots?

4.1.39 请船长放心，我们每一位引航员都是在引航站确认健康的前提下，才被派来执行引航任务的。

Don't worry, Mr. Captain, local pilot station will only send healthy pilots on board.

4.1.40 非常感谢你的支持与配合，敬请关注引航员提供的最新疫情信息，中国引航始终为你提供专业、一流的引航服务。

Thank you very much for your support and cooperation. You can get the latest epidemic information from pilots, Chinese pilots will always provide you with professional and first-class pilotage service.

4.1.41 我船满载防疫物资。

My ship is fully loaded with anti-epidemic materials.

4.1.42 中国加油！

Stay strong, China!

4.1.43 船长，因为大雾我被要求驻船。

Mr. Captain, I have to stay on board because of the heavy fog.

4.1.44 船长，可以给我提供引航员房间么？

Mr. Captain, would you please provide a pilot cabin for me?

4.1.45 船长，引航员的房间做过清洁和消毒吗？

Did someone clean and disinfect the pilot's cabin, Mr. Captain?

4.1.46 船长，可以给我提供一套新的寝具么？

Mr. Captain, would you please offer me a new bedding?

4.1.47 谢谢你船长，我不需要咖啡，如果可以，请为我准备一瓶矿泉水。

Thank you, Mr. Captain, I do not drink coffee, Please give me a bottle of mineral water if available.

4.1.48 我可以在引航员房间用餐么？

Could I have my meal in pilot cabin?

4.1.49 餐食准备好了后，服务员会将餐食给送到引航员房间的。你可以放心所有的餐具都是彻底消毒过的。

The steward will bring your meal to pilot cabin when it is ready. All the tableware have been sterilized thoroughly.

4.1.50 船长，请确保食物被完全煮熟（尤其是肉和动物产品）。

Mr. Captain, please make sure the food is fully cooked

(especially for meat and animal products).

4.1.51 船长，请理解。我自带食物没有别的意思，这是为我和你船人员的健康和安全着想。

Please don't mind, Mr. Captain. I bring my own food on board for the health and safety of both your crew and me.

4.1.52 引航员，你带着便携式酒精消毒剂么？如果没有，我们可以提供。

Mr. Pilot, do you have alcohol disinfectant with you? If not, we can provide it for you.

4.1.53 如果你有什么需要，请拨打驾驶台电话。

If you need anything, please call the bridge.

4.1.54 引航员，如果你需要去驾驶台或者甲板，请拨打驾驶台电话，会有驾驶员陪同并给你带路。

Mr. Pilot, if you need to go to the bridge or the deck, please call the bridge. There will be an officer accompanying with you.

4.1.55 我会一直开着甚高频对讲机与护航拖船保持联系的。如有任何紧急情况发生，请马上通知我。

I will keep in touch with the escort tugboat by VHF at

all times. In case of any emergency, please notify me immediately.

4.2 检疫常用语句

Frequently used sentences in quarantine inspection

4.2.1 船长，请把检疫所需文件都准备好。
Mr. Captain, please get all your documents ready for the quarantine inspection.

4.2.2 船长，请问你知道新冠肺炎吗?
Mr. Captain, have you ever heard COVID-19?

4.2.3 我们从国际海事组织关于新冠肺炎疫情报告4204 和 4203 的通函里收到的消息。
We have got the IMO Circulars (Nos 4203 and 4204) on COVID-19 outbreak.

4.2.4 请问船上人员身体状况都健康吗?
Are all persons on board in good health?

4.2.5 你船上有人发烧 / 咳嗽吗?
Does anybody have a fever/cough on board?

4.2.6 我船上没有人员有发热 / 咳嗽症状。

No one on board has a fever/cough.

4.2.7 你船针对新冠肺炎进行消毒了吗?

Have you disinfected your ship to prevent COVID-19?

4.2.8 请问船舶在停靠港口前,是否对驾驶台、生活区等公共区域消毒?

Did you disinfect the bridge, the accommodation area and other public areas before entering the port?

4.2.9 船上配有的口罩已经发放给船员,足够本港使用。

Each crew member has got enough face masks for this port.

4.2.10 为了你和他人的健康,并避免交叉感染风险,请佩戴口罩。

Please wear a face mask for the health of others and yourself.

4.2.11 请问船员下地是否需要佩戴口罩?

Does my crew need to wear a mask when going ashore?

4.2.12 疫情期间,我建议,船员避免下地或与外来

人员接触。

During the outbreak of the epidemic, I suggest all crew avoid going ashore or any unnecessary contact with visitors.

4.2.13 请问船上是否对船员进行过疫情相关知识及防疫措施的培训?

Have you ever conducted any training of epidemic knowledge and precautionary measures on board to prevent COVID-19?

4.2.14 船上为本次疫情准备了什么个人防护用品? 是否随时可用? 是否都处于良好的状态? 船员是否接受过正规的防护用品穿戴培训? 要知道个人防护措施远比在空中喷洒消毒剂有效果。

What kind of personal protective equipment do you have on board? Are they available at any time? Are they in good condition? Have the crew received any training on wearing personal protective equipment properly? You know that personal preventive measures are far more effective than disinfecting in the air.

4.2.15 请问有船员被新冠病毒感染吗?

Have any crew been infected with COVID-19？

4.2.16　船上无人染疫。请问有码头工人感染新冠病毒吗？

No one is infected with COVID-19. Has any stevedore been infected with COVID-19?

4.2.17　目前没有发现码头工人感染新冠病毒，所有码头工人上船前都会经过体温检测。

None of the stevedores has been found infected with COVID-19. All of them will have their body temperatures checked before boarding the ship.

4.2.18　船舶在港口停留期间，船员有被新冠病毒感染的可能吗？

Is there any possibility for crew to be infected with COVID-19 during the port stay?

4.2.19　有被感染的可能，但是概率很低，目前本港没有发生船员在港口停留期间被新冠病毒感染的案例。

There is a possibility of infection, but the risk is very low. So far, no crew members has been infected during the port stay.

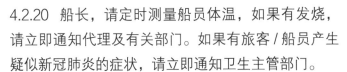
4.2.20 船长，请定时测量船员体温，如果有发烧，请立即通知代理及有关部门。如果有旅客/船员产生疑似新冠肺炎的症状，请立即通知卫生主管部门。

Mr. Captain, please check the temperature of the crew at a certain time of the day. If anyone has a fever, please inform your agent and relevant departments immediately. If any passenger/crew is suspected to be infected with COVID-19, you must make a report to the public health authorities immediately.

4.2.21 我怀疑有一位旅客/船员被感染了，出现了……症状，靠泊后需要医疗援助。目前旅客/船员的病情稳定。

There is a suspected case of COVID-19 on board. One passenger/crew has symptoms like…,and we need medical assistance right after berthing. The passenger/crew is in a stable condition so far.

4.2.22 对于防止感染新冠病毒，你们有根据 IMO 通函采取过什么预防措施吗？

Have you taken any precautionary measures in accordance with the IMO circulars to prevent COVID-19?

4.2.23 你们船上有没有成立船舶疫情防控工作组？

Have you set up a working group for epidemic prevention and control on board?

4.2.24　你船有专门收集废弃的新冠病毒防护用品的垃圾桶吗?

Do you have a garbage bin designated for collecting used protective items?

4.2.25　你船有足够的防护用品（如口罩、手套、护目镜、防护服）吗?

Do you have enough protective equipment (such as face masks, gloves, goggles and protective suits) on board?

4.2.26　船长，你们船上有设立单独的紧急隔离房间吗? 该房间位置是否远离餐厅、驾驶台、集控室等人员密集地?

Mr. Captain, is there any separate room for emergency isolation? Is the room far away from the dining room, bridge, engine control room or other public areas?

4.2.27　我们的船员都佩戴了口罩、护目镜和手套。

All of our crew are wearing face masks, safety goggles and gloves.

4.2.28　你船每天对全体船员做体温检测和记录吗？

Do you check temperature for all crew members and record everyday?

4.2.29 船长应该在进港前报告里面报告健康情况。请问代理有给你发中华人民共和国出入境健康申明卡吗？所有船员都已经如实填写并签名了吗？请将出入境健康申明卡准备好，以便靠港之后等待检疫官员的检查。

The master should report the health condition of all crew before entering the port. Did the agent send you the exit/entry Health Declaration Form of the People's Republic of China? Have all crew members filled in their form properly with signature? Please prepare the exit/entry health declaration form, and wait for the inspection carried out by the quarantine officers after berthing.

4.2.30 你船在靠港期间是否采取了足够的防护措施？
Did you take sufficient preventive measures during the port stay?

4.2.31 船长，能让我测一下你的体温吗？
Mr. Captain, may I check your temperature?

4.2.32 请问你船之前14天停靠的港口有无船员下地？

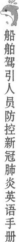
Would you please tell me if any crew went ashore in the previous ports of call within 14 days?

4.2.33 在今日之前 14 天的靠港期间，有没有外来人员有发热或者咳嗽的情况发生？

During the previous ports of call in the last 14 days, did any visitors have a fever or coughs?

4.2.34 在挂靠该港口期间，有无该国的检疫官员对你船进行过检疫？

Did any quarantine officer inspect the ship during the port stay?

4.2.35 最近 30 天是否更换过船员？若有，在哪一港发生？换班船员来自哪里？你了解他们的行程吗？

Is there any crew change in the past 30 days? If so, where did it happen? Where did new crew members come from? Do you have any idea of their travel history?

4.2.36 更换的新船员是否有来自疫情高发国家或者地区的？

Are the new crew from the epicentre countries or regions?

4.2.37 换班船员来自菲律宾，他们乘飞机从马尼拉至新加坡，之后乘交通艇到锚地换班。

The new crew members came from the Philippines. They came to Singapore from Manila by air, and then they came on board by a traffic boat when the vessel anchored in that port.

4.2.38 由于换班船员途经了 A 国，且换班时间小于 14 日，你的靠港计划要等待检疫部门通过后再确定。

As the new crew members travelled through A and it is less than 14 days , your berthing schedule cannot be confirmed without permission from the quarantine department.

4.2.39 你船是从 A 国来的，请问有没有采取有效的防护及消毒措施？

Your ship came from A. Have you taken proper protection and disinfection measures?

4.2.40 你船在 A 国靠港期间与外来人员有过接触吗？

Did any crew contact with visitors during the port stay in A?

4.2.41 船长，上一港（A 国）现在疫情较重，在那是否有船员下过地？

Mr. Captain, there is a severe epidemic in country A. Is

there any crew went ashore there?

4.2.42 据你船报告，在停靠上一港时有船员感染了新冠病毒，这就是我们必须采取特别防护措施的原因。

According to your report, some crew were infected with COVID-19 at your last port of call. That is why we have to take special precautions for your vessel.

4.2.43 非常感谢，我们理解并会遵守港口的相关规定。

Thank you very much, we understood and will comply with the relevant port regulations.

4.2.44 核酸检测结果为阳性 / 阴性。

The nucleic acid test result is positive/negative.

4.2.45 根据检查结果，你的船舶需要接受熏蒸消毒。

According to the inspection results, we will apply fumigation to disinfect your vessel.

4.2.46 熏蒸的工作人员将提供你一份检查表以供参考。

Fumigation operators will provide one checklist for your reference.

4.2.47 你认为我们的检疫合格了吗?

Do you think we are qualified for free pratique?

4.2.48 船长，我们对你船所做的防疫工作很满意。你船是合格的，这是入境许可证，现在你可以降下检疫旗了。

Mr. Captain, we are satisfied with what you have done for the quarantine job. Here is your entry permit. You could haul down the quarantine flag now.

4.3 移民检查

Immigration inspection

4.3.1 船长，请通知所有船员到会议室来接受检查，检查时船员需要佩戴口罩，保持至少 1.5m 的安全距离。

Mr. Captain. Please call all crew members to the conference room for the immigration inspection. Don't forget to remind them to wear face masks and keep a safe distance forat least 1.5 meters.

4.3.2 我马上通知。

I will call them to the conference room right now.

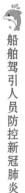

4.3.3 虽然你船申请了本航次的登岸证，但非常遗憾地通知你，由于新冠肺炎的缘故，所有船员必须留在船上。

Although your vessel had applied for the shore pass for this voyage visit, we are sorry to inform you that all crew must stay on board because of current pandemic situation of COVID-19.

4.3.4 船长，这是关于预防新冠肺炎的告知书，请所有船员知悉。

Mr. Captain. This is a notification about the prevention of COVID-19. Please inform all your crew.

4.4 港口当局检查
Harbour authority inspection

4.4.1 船长，下午好！可以给我看一下你船制定的疫情防控管理计划吗？

Good afternoon, Mr. Captain. Could you show me your prevention plan for COVID-19?

4.4.2 这个计划是根据国际海事组织通告和新冠肺炎指南并且特别为保护船员健康而制定的。

The plan is based on the IMO circulars and guidelines of preventing COVID-19 and is specifically designed to protect the health of crew members.

4.4.3 你船应对新冠肺炎的管理计划和实施记录很完备，我们相信你船对新冠肺炎有很好的防护措施，现在让我们开始安全检查。

After reviewing your management plan and implementation records for preventing COVID-19, we believe that you have perfectly implemented the protective measures. Now we can start the safety inspection.

4.4.4 船长，我们已经完成对你船的安全检查，全部符合 PSC 的要求。虽然目前正处于新冠肺炎疫情期，但我们希望你们在港愉快。

Mr. Captain, we have completed the safety inspection for your vessel and the result shows that your vessel meets all the PSC's requirements. We hope you enjoy your stay at this port , though we are facing a challenging time of COVID-19 outbreak.

4.4.5 港口有什么应对新冠肺炎疫情的措施需要我们船员配合的?

Are there any measures for COVID-19 from the port

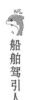

authority that requires the cooperation of our crew?

4.4.6 所有进出港口人员必须测量体温，体温正常的方可进出。

All personnel entering or leaving port must have their body temperature checked first. They cannot enter or leave the port unless their body temperatures are normal.

4.4.7 所有的入境船舶，检疫官员都将登船测量船员体温，并进行其他健康检查。

For all inbound ships, quarantine officers will board the ship to take crew members' body temperature and conduct other health checks.

4.4.8 所有船员都需要填写健康申明卡。无特殊情况，禁止船员更换和上岸。

All crew members must fill in the Health Declaration Form. Generally, replacement and disembarkation of crew will be prohibited.

4.4.9 请尽量避免在本港安排船舶物料供应，以减少人员交叉感染概率。如有船舶必须补充供给物资，务必提前向港方申报。

Try not to arrange provision supplies on board at this port to reduce cross infection. If you have to, you shall apply to the port authority in advance.

4.4.10 所有船舶在泊期间，需要安排专人在梯口值守，防止无关人员上下船舶，并对所有上下船的人员进行体温测量和登记。

During the port stay, a designated crew shall be assigned on the gangway to prevent irrelevant people from boarding. He will also check and record the temperature of all who embark or disembark the ship.

4.4.11 凡装载有防疫物资的船舶，请告知船公司及代理提前做好申报，提供具体船名、航次、箱号、排号等信息，我们将安排绿色通道，第一时间安排进出港及接卸作业。

For ships carrying epidemic protective materials, please inform your shipping company and agents to make declarations by providing information including the ship's name, voyage number, and container numbers and locations in advance. Port authorities will offer the ship priority service, and arrange berthing schedule and cargo operating as soon as possible.

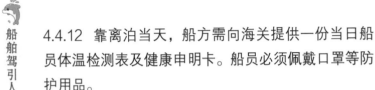

4.4.12 靠离泊当天，船方需向海关提供一份当日船员体温检测表及健康申明卡。船员必须佩戴口罩等防护用品。

On the day of berthing and unberthing, a copy of crew members' temperature records for that day and Health Declaration Forms should be provided to the Customs. All crew should wear protective equipment such as face masks.

4.4.13 建议取消船员更换，如果一定需要更换，必须检测过船员的体温并做好记录。

It is recommended to cancel any crew change. If really necessary, check and record crew members' temperatures.

4.4.14 船舶在抵达报告线时，应向交管中心报告并申请靠泊计划。同时，应将船上人员及旅客的体温情况向交管中心做简单说明。

When arriving at the reporting line, captain should make a report to the VTS and apply for a berthing schedule. At the same time, captain shall make a brief report about the body temperatures of all crew and passengers to the VTS as well.

4.4.15 如船上人员及旅客的体温异常，交管中心将安排船舶直接到锚地锚泊，等候检疫确认。

If anyone has a fever on board, the VTS should instruct the ship to proceed to the anchorage area directly and wait for quarantine inspection.

4.4.16 所有船舶靠泊后，非生产需要，禁止将舷梯放下。

After berthing, it is forbidden to lower the gangway unless there is a need for necessary cargo operation.

4.4.17 原则上不允许船员下船，不安排船员换班、外部人员访船及公司检查等。

In principle, crew are not allowed to disembark. Try to avoid the crew change, ship visiting and internal inspections during the port stay.

4.5 梯口值班

Gangway watch

4.5.1 船上正在办理检疫手续，暂时不允许人员上下船，必须等检疫合格获得许可，我才能放下舷梯，请稍等。

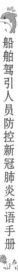

When the ship is undergoing a quarantine inspection, people are not allowed to board the ship. I can't lower the gangway until we are free of pratique. Please wait a moment.

4.5.2 代理你好，请戴好口罩。在船上请与其他人保持 1.5 m 以上安全距离。

Hi! Mr. Agent, please wear your face mask. You should keep a distance for at least 1.5 meters away from other people onboard.

4.5.3 代理，我需要测量一下你的体温。

Mr. Agent, I need to check your temperature.

4.5.4 体温 36.5℃，很好。请出示你的证件。

36.5 degrees Celsius, great. Please show me your ID.

4.5.5 请填一下登船记录，写下你的姓名、联系方式、登船目的并签名。

Please fill in the boarding record, write down your name, contact information, purpose of boarding, and sign here.

4.5.6 请稍等，我将安排专门人员引导你到指定区域办理相关手续，大副将在那儿等你。

Wait a moment please. I will arrange a special crew to guide you to the designated area for relevant procedures, and our chief mate will be waiting for you there.

4.6 介绍疫情常用语句
Frequently used sentences about the epidemic

4.6.1 引航员，你好！中国的疫情现状如何？
Hello, Mr. Pilot. How is the epidemic situation in China?

4.6.2 船长，你好！中国政府对新冠肺炎采取了强有力的防治措施，目前疫情已经得到了有效控制。
Hello, Mr. Captain, the Chinese government has taken effective measures to control the spread of COVID-19 and has already kept the epidemic under control.

4.6.3 我们的港口是十分安全的，目前没有发现新冠肺炎病例。
Our port is very safe and no confirmed case of COVID-19 is found so far.

4.6.4 我们省 / 市 / 港口已连续 5 天没有新增疑似和确诊病例了。

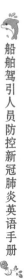
Our province/city/port has no new suspected or confirmed cases of COVID-19 for 5 consecutive days.

4.6.5 这个港口／城市的新冠肺炎疫情不是很严重，疑似病例和确诊病例每天都在减少，截至目前没有死亡病例。相关部门在交通管制和控制人员流动方面都采取了积极有效的措施，很好地控制了疫情的扩散。

The situation of COVID-19 at this port/city is not serious. The number of suspected and confirmed cases is declining every day, and there is no death caused by the virus for the time being. Relevant authorities have been taking strict and effective measures in traffic control and movement of people at all times. As a result, the spread of the epidemic has been well controlled.

4.6.6 疫情在中国已经得到有效的控制，但是全球疫情却在恶化。

The epidemic has already been effectively controlled in China recently, but it gets worse in some other parts of the world.

4.6.7 船员们每天都关注疫情变化的新闻吗？

Did crew members follow the updated news of the

epidemic every day?

4.6.8　A 国近日新增 161 例新冠肺炎确诊病例。

Country A has confirmed 161 new cases of COVID-19 recently.

4.6.9　A 国和 B 国进入了爆发高峰期。

A and B are at the peak of the outbreak.

4.6.10　我认为 A 国和 B 国可以借鉴中国经验，及早采取措施。

I think A and B could learn something from China's experience and take measures as early as possible.

4.6.11　即使本月底一切可以恢复正常，我们仍然建议多佩戴一段时间的口罩。

Even if everything may return to normal at the end of this month, it is still recommended to wear face masks for a longer time.

4.6.12　你船上的船员对新型冠状病毒的传播方式和途径有所了解吗？

Do your crew know anything about the transmission methods and routes of the SARS-CoV-2?

4.6.13 这种病毒的传染能力非常强，会通过飞沫、接触等方式传播。

The virus is highly contagious and can spread through droplets and contact.

4.6.14 在医疗资源相对缺乏的时候，人员隔离、专业处置、减少交叉感染是防止疫情扩散的有效手段。

When medical resources are relatively scarce, isolation, professional treatment and reduction of cross infection are effective means to prevent the spread of the epidemic.

4.6.15 保持强健体魄、充足精力和乐观态度，做好个人清洁消毒卫生，审慎对待疫情，减少外出，或许是目前最有效的解决方法。

Being robust, energetic and optimistic, practising high standards of personal hygiene, treating the outbreak rationally, and reducing the frequency of going out might be the most effective prevention solution at present.

4.6.16 所有确诊病例必须在指定医院隔离治疗。

All confirmed cases must be isolated and treated in a designated hospital.

4.6.17 请相信我们会提供最及时和完善的医疗服务。

Please believe that we will provide the most timely and best medical services.

4.6.18 因为出现"假阴性"检测结果，核酸检测需要多测几次。

Repeated nucleic acid tests are necessary, since false negative results have been reported.

4.6.19 新冠病毒传播扩散很快，而且疫苗和特效药尚未研制出来，目前已对多国造成威胁，为了船上人员安全健康，我们采取防范措施是必要的。

The spread of SARS-CoV-2 is extremely fast, vaccines and medicines against the virus have not yet been developed. At present, it has posed a threat to many countries. For the safety and health of crew members on board, it is necessary to take precautions.

4.6.20 船长先生，请你们一定要多加小心，认真对待这次疫情，对于有疑似症状的船员一定要第一时间采取隔离并向相关部门汇报。

Mr. Captain, please be more careful and take the epidemic seriously. Any crew member with suspected symptoms must be isolated immediately, and the master should report to relevant organizations as soon as possible.

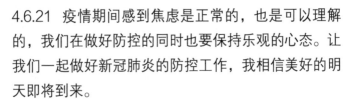

4.6.21 疫情期间感到焦虑是正常的，也是可以理解的，我们在做好防控的同时也要保持乐观的心态。让我们一起做好新冠肺炎的防控工作，我相信美好的明天即将到来。

It is normal and understandable to feel anxious during the epidemic outbreak, but we should keep an optimistic attitude to prevent and control the spread of the virus. Let's work together to fight against COVID-19. I believe that a bright tomorrow is coming soon.

第5章 疫情现状
Chapter 5
Epidemic Situation

5.1 中国目前的疫情状况（截至 2020 年 3 月 22 日）
The latest coronavirus epidemic situation in China (as of March 22nd, 2020)

3 月 22 日 0—24 时，31 个省（自治区、直辖市）和新疆生产建设兵团报告新增确诊病例 39 例，均为境外输入病例，新增死亡病例 9 例（湖北 9 例），新增疑似病例 47 例。

全国现有确诊病例 5120 例（其中重症病例 1749 例），累计治愈出院病例 72703 例，累计死亡病例 3270 例，累计报告确诊病例 81093 例，现有疑似病例 136 例。累计追踪到密切接触者 688993 人，尚在医学观察的密切接触者 10701 人。（信息来源：国家卫生健康委员会官方网站 http://www.nhc.gov.cn/xcs/yqtb/202003/fbd8871d80574991a4913cd180f83402.shtml）

On March 22, 39 new confirmed cases (all of which were imported from overseas), 9 new deaths (all in Hubei Province) and 47 new suspected cases were reported nationwide.

As of March 22, the number of confirmed cases in China was 5,120 (including 1,749 critical patients) and the number of suspected cases was 136.The cumulative number of patients cured and discharged was 72,703, the cumulative number of deaths caused by COVID-19 was 3,270, and the cumulative number of confirmed case was 81,093.The number of traced close contact was 688,993, including 10,701 close contacts were still under medical observation. (Source: *Official Website of National Health Commission of the People's Republic of China* http://www.nhc.gov.cn/xcs/yqtb/202003/fbd8871 d80574991a4913cd180f83402.shtml)

5.2 中国防控疫情的措施(截至2020年3月22日) China's prevention and control measures of COVID-19 (as of March 22nd, 2020)

5.2.1 经中央军委主席习近平批准，军队抽组1400名医护人员于2月3日起承担武汉火神山新冠肺炎专科医院医疗救治任务。火神山医院主要救治确诊患者，编设床位1000张。(信息来源:《中国日报双语新闻》https://mp.weixin.qq.com/s/kw-

N8yPqdAOwn5NJj7anbw）

Approved by Xi Jinping, Chairman of the Central Military Commission (CPC), 1,400 military medical staff are tasked with treating patients in Huoshenshan Hospital in Wuhan starting from Feburary 3. Huoshenshan Hospital, with a capacity of 1,000 beds, is a makeshift hospital dedicated to treating patients infected with COVID-19. (Source: *People's Daily* https://mp.weixin.qq.com/s/kw-N8yPqdAOwn5NJj7anbw)

5.2.2 2 月 25 日，国务院应对新型冠状病毒肺炎疫情联防联控机制发布《关于依法科学精准做好新冠肺炎疫情防控工作的通知》，通知明确要求，对疫情特别严重的湖北省继续采取最严格的防控措施，已实施交通管控的武汉市和湖北省其他地市，严控人员输出。（信息来源：《中国日报双语新闻》https://mp.weixin.qq.com/s/n0PiGkWYo3WYjzuBlwC5jQ）

The Joint Prevention and Control Mechanism of the State Council issued *Notice on Scientific and Accurate Prevention and Control of COVID-19 Outbreak* on February 25. It requests that Hubei province, the most severe epicentre of the outbreak in China, continues to take the most stringent prevention and control measures.

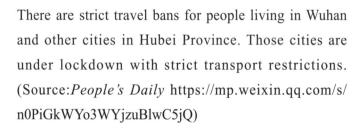

There are strict travel bans for people living in Wuhan and other cities in Hubei Province. Those cities are under lockdown with strict transport restrictions. (Source:*People's Daily* https://mp.weixin.qq.com/s/n0PiGkWYo3WYjzuBlwC5jQ)

5.2.3 3月5日，交通运输部海事局印发紧急通知，要求各级海事管理机构全力做好疫情内防扩散、外防输入工作，建立与当地政府、口岸卫生检疫部门的应急联络机制，落实各项联防联控措施，切实做好口岸疫情防控工作。（信息来源：中国交通新闻网 http://www.zgjtb.com/2020-03/10/content-238299.htm）

On March 5, the Maritime Safety Administration of the Ministry of Transport issued an emergency notice, requiring the maritime administrative agencies at all levels to make all-out efforts to prevent both imported cases and spread within the city.An emergency liaison mechanism shall be established with the local government and port health and quarantine departments to implement various joint prevention and control measures, and effective measures at port shall be taken to prevent and control the epidemic.(Source: http://www.zgjtb.com/2020-03/10/content-238299.htm)

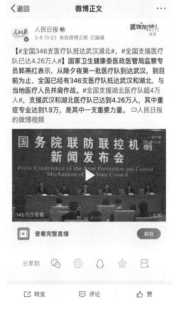

5.2.4 3月8日，国家卫生健康委医政医管局监察专员郭燕红在国务院联防联控机制举行的发布会上介绍，截至当日，全国有346支医疗队，共计4.26万人抵达武汉和湖北，与当地的医务人员一起并肩作战，全力开展医疗救治工作，有效提高治愈率，降低病亡率。（信息来源：人民日报微博：https://m.weibo.cn/2803301701/4480224555686117）

Guo Yanhong, a supervision commissioner from Medical Administration of the National Health Commission said on a press conference of the Joint Prevention and Control Mechanism of the State Council: 346 medical teams nationwide, with a total of 42,600 doctors and nurses, have arrived in Wuhan by March 8th and are fighting together with the local medical professionals. They would try their best to enhance the recovery rate and decrease the mortality rate. (Source: *People's Daily weibo*)

5.2.5 为帮助航运公司妥善解决疫情期间船员换班困难问题，3月12日交通运输部和人力资源社会保障部联合发布公告，指导航运公司做好中国籍国际航行船舶在船船员换班工作，保障船舶正常运营，保护船员劳动权益。（信息来源：中华人民共和国海事局官方网站 https://www.msa.gov.cn/page/article.do?articleId=6C12DE10-23EA-457A-AE97-F53380F2169F）

In order to help the shipping companies to solve the problem of crew shift properly during the outbreak, on March 12, the Ministry of Transport and the Ministry of Human Resources and Social Security jointly issued a notice to guide shipping companies to exchange crew for Chinese ships on international routes, ensuring the operation of vessels and protecting labor rights and interests of the crew.(Source: *China MSA Official Website* https://www.msa.gov.cn/page/article.do?articleId=6C12DE10-23EA-457A-AE97-F53380F2169F)

5.2.6 3月16日，最高人民法院、最高人民检察院、公安部、司法部、海关总署联合发布《关于进一步加强国境卫生检疫工作 依法惩治妨害国境卫生检疫违法犯罪的意见》。根据《意见》，对检疫传染病染疫人或者染疫嫌疑人拒绝隔离、不如实填报健康申明卡等，有引起鼠疫、霍乱、黄热病以及新冠肺炎等国务院确定和公布的其他检疫传染病传播或者有传播严重危险的，以妨害国境卫生检疫罪定罪处罚。（信息来源：央广新闻微信公众号 http://www.chinanews.com/sh/2020/03-16/9127211.shtml）

On March 16, the Supreme People's Court, the Supreme People's Procuratorate, the Ministry of Public Security, the Ministry of Justice and the General Administration of Customs jointly issued the *Opinions on Further Strengthening Frontier Health and Quarantine Work in Punishing Illegal Crimes that Stifled Frontier Health and Quarantine* (hereinafter referred to as "Opinions"). According to the "Opinions", anyone who refuses to quarantine or fails to fill in the Health Declaration Form truthfully, or spreads diseases identified and announced by the State Council, such as plague, cholera, yellow fever and COVID-19, shall be convicted and punished for the crime of obstructing frontier health and quarantine work. (Source: *Central Radio and Television Station*

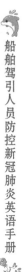

WeChat Official Account http://www.chinanews.com/sh/2020/03-16/9127211.shtml)

5.2.7 3月22日，民航局、外交部、国家卫生健康委员会、海关总署、国家移民管理局等五部门发布公告表示，自3月23日零时（北京时间）开始，所有目的地为北京的国际始发客运航班均须从天津、石家庄、太原、呼和浩特、上海浦东、济南、青岛、南京、沈阳、大连、郑州、西安12个指定的第一入境点入境。（信息来源：中国民航网 http://www.caacnews.com.cn/1/1/202003/t20200322-1296265.html）

On March 22, the Civil Aviation Administration, the Ministry of Foreign Affairs, National Health Commission, the General Administration of Customs, National Immigration Administration announced that starting from March 23, all international passenger flights with Beijing as the destination should enter China from 12 designated first ports of entry including Tianjin, Shijiazhuang, Taiyuan, Hohhot, Shanghai Pudong, Jinan, Shenyang, Dalian, Qingdao, Nanjing, Zhengzhou and Xi'an. (Source: *CAAC News* http://www.caacnews.com.cn/1/1/202003/t20200322-1296265.html)

附录一：常用词汇
Appendix I : Vocabulary

aerosol['eərəsɒl] 气溶胶

asymptomatic [ˌeɪsɪmptə'mætɪk] 无症状的

axillary [æk'sɪlərɪ] 腋下

bacteria [bæk'tɪərɪə] 细菌

clinic ['klɪnɪk] 门诊

coronavirus [kəˌrəunə'vaɪərəs] 冠状病毒

designated ['dezɪgˌneɪtɪd] 指定的

diagnosis [ˌdaɪəg'nəʊsɪs] 诊断

diarrhea [ˌdaɪəˌrɪə] 腹泻

dishware['dɪʃweə] 餐具

disinfectant [ˌdɪsɪn'fektənt] 消毒剂

droplet ['drɒplət] 飞沫

dyspnea [dɪsp'ni:ə] 呼吸困难

elbow ['elbəʊ] 肘部

electrolyte [ɪ'lektrəlaɪt] 电解质

emergency[ɪ'mɜ:dʒənsi] 突发事件

epidemic[ˌepɪ'demɪk] 疫情

epidemiology [ˌepɪˌdi:mi'ɒlədʒi] 流行病学

exposure[ɪkˈspəʊʒə(r)] 暴露

(face) mask [mɑːsk] 口罩

fatality[fəˈtæləti] 死亡

fatigue [fəˈtiːg] 乏力

fibrosis [faɪˈbrəʊsɪs] 纤维化

goggles[ˈɡɒɡls] 护目镜

guarantee [ˌɡærənˈtiː] 确保

guidance[ˈɡaɪdns] 指导

immunity[ɪˈmjuːnəti] 免疫力

incubation [ˌɪŋkjʊˈbeɪʃn] 潜伏期

infection[ɪnˈfekʃn] 感染

isolation[ˈaɪsəleɪt] 隔离

monitor[ˈmɒnɪtə(r)] 监控

negative[ˈneɡətɪv] 【医】阴性的

nausea [ˈnɔːziə] 恶心

morbidity [mɔːˈbɪdəti] 发病率

mortality [mɔːˈtæləti] 死亡率

nucleic[njuːˈkliːɪk] 核酸

palpitation [ˌpælpɪˈteɪʃ(ə)n] 心慌

pandemic [pænˈdemɪk] （全国或全球性）流行病

pneumonia[njuːˈməʊniə] 肺炎

positive[ˈpɒzətɪv] 【医】阳性的

recommended [ˌrekəˈmendɪd] 推荐的

release [rɪˈliːs] 解除隔离

respiratory[rəˈspɪrətri; ˈrespərətri] 呼吸的

rumor [ˈruːmə] 谣言

serodiagnosis [ˌsɪərəʊdaɪəˈgnəʊsɪs] 血清诊断

sneeze[sniːz] 打喷嚏

surgical [ˈsɜːdʒɪkl] 外科的

suspected[səˈspektɪd] 疑似的

vaccine[ˈvæksiːn] 疫苗

常用短语：附录二
Appendix Ⅱ：Phrases

84 disinfectant 84 消毒液

ARDS（AcuteRespiratory Distress Syndrome）急性呼吸窘迫综合征

aerosol transmission 气溶胶传播

air circulation 空气循环

antiviral drug 抗病毒药

CDC（Centers for Disease Control and Prevention）疾病预防和控制中心

clinical manifestation 临床表现

close contact 密切接触者

common cold 普通感冒

confirmed case 确诊病例

contact transmission 接触传播

COVID-19（Coronavirus Disease 2019）新型冠状病毒肺炎（简称：新冠肺炎）

cross infection 交叉感染

death toll 死亡人数

designated hospital 定点医院

droplet transmission 飞沫传播

dry cough 干咳

epidemic area 疫区

epidemiological investigation 流行病学调查

exogenous infection 外源性感染

fatality rate 致死率

fever clinic 发热门诊

gastrointestinal discomfort 胃肠道不适

health authorities 卫生主管部门

health declaration form 健康申明卡

incubation/ latent period 潜伏期

kidney failure 肾（功能）衰竭

medical assistance 医疗援助

medical institution 医疗机构

MSA（Maritime Safety Administration） 海事局

mucous membrane 黏膜

nasal obstruction 鼻塞

NHC（National Health Commission）国家卫生健康委员会

protective clothing 防护服

protective gloves 防护手套

preventive measure 预防措施

quarantine department 检疫部门

quarantine officer 检疫官

respiratory diseases 呼吸道疾病（呼吸系统疾病）

SARS-CoV-2（Severe Acute Respiratory Syndrome Coronavirus 2）新型冠状病毒

septic shock 脓毒症性休克

shortness of breath; panting 呼吸急促（气促）

surgical mask 外科口罩

suspected case 疑似病例

temperature detection 体温检测

WHO（World Health Organization）世界卫生组织

附录三：健康申明卡
Appendix Ⅲ : Health Declaration Form

中华人民共和国
出／入境健康申明卡

请在相应"□"中划"√"　　　　　　　　　　　　　　　　　□出境　□入境

姓名：＿＿＿＿＿＿＿　性别：□男　□女　出生日期：＿＿＿＿＿　年＿＿＿＿月＿＿＿＿日国

籍（地区）：＿＿＿＿＿＿＿＿＿　常驻城市：＿＿＿＿＿＿＿＿＿　职业：＿＿＿＿＿＿

1. 证件类型：□护照　□前往港澳通行证　□往来台湾通行证　□往来港澳通行证

　　□港澳居民来往内地通行证　□台湾居民来往大陆通行证　□中华人民共和国出入境通行证

　　□其它证件：＿＿＿＿＿＿＿＿＿＿＿＿　证件号码：＿＿＿＿＿＿＿＿＿

　　航班（船班／车次）号：＿＿＿＿＿＿＿＿　座位号：＿＿＿＿＿＿＿＿＿

　　出／入境口岸：＿＿＿＿＿＿＿＿＿　出／入境目的地：＿＿＿＿＿＿＿＿

2. □境内／□境外有效手机号或其它联系方式：＿＿＿＿＿＿＿＿＿＿＿＿＿＿＿＿＿＿＿＿

　　其它境内有效联系人及联系方式：＿＿＿＿＿＿＿＿＿＿＿＿＿＿＿＿＿＿＿＿＿＿

　　自今日起后 14 日的住址（请详细填写，境内住址请具体到街道／社区及门牌号或宾馆

　　地　址）：＿＿＿＿＿＿＿＿＿＿＿＿＿＿＿＿＿＿＿＿＿＿＿＿＿＿＿＿＿＿＿＿

　　＿＿＿＿＿＿＿＿＿＿＿＿＿＿＿＿＿＿＿＿＿＿＿＿＿＿＿＿＿＿＿＿＿＿＿＿＿

　　如果属于因公来华（归国），请填写邀请方：＿＿＿＿＿＿＿　接待方：＿＿＿＿＿＿

3. 过去 14 日内，您在中国旅行或居住的省（自治区、直辖市）和／或港澳台地区（请具体到城

　　市）：＿＿＿＿＿＿＿＿＿＿＿＿＿＿＿＿＿＿＿＿＿＿＿＿＿＿＿＿＿＿＿＿＿＿＿

4. 过去 14 日内，您旅行或居住的国家和地区：＿＿＿＿＿＿＿＿＿＿＿＿＿＿＿＿＿＿＿

　　过去 14 日内，曾接触新冠肺炎确诊病例／疑似病例／无症状感染者　　　　□是 □否

　　过去 14 日内，曾接触有发热和／或呼吸道症状的患者　　　　　　　　　　□是 □否

　　过去 14 日内，所居住社区曾报告有新冠肺炎病例　　　　　　　　　　　　□是 □否

　　过去 14 日内，所在办公室／家庭等是否出现 2 人及以上有发热和／或呼吸道症状

　　　　　　　　　　　　　　　　　　　　　　　　　　　　　　　　　　　　□是 □否

5. 过去 14 日内和或出／入境时，是否有以下症状：　　　　　　　　　　　　□是 □否

　　如勾选"是"，请选择□发热　□寒战　□干咳　□咳痰　□鼻塞　□流涕　□咽痛　□头痛

　　□乏力口头晕　□肌肉酸痛　□关节酸痛　□气促　□呼吸困难　□胸闷　□胸痛　□结膜充血口恶心

　　□呕吐　□腹泻　□腹痛　□其它症状＿＿＿＿＿＿＿＿＿＿＿＿＿＿＿＿

　　过去 14 日内，是否曾服用退烧药、感冒药、止咳药　　　　　　　　　　　□是 □否

6. 过去 14 日内，如果您曾接受新型冠状病毒检测，则检测结果是否为阳性　　□是 □否

尊敬的出入境人员，根据有关法律法规规定，为了您和他人健康，请如实逐项填报，如有隐瞒或虚假填报，

将依照《中华人民共和国国境卫生检疫法》追究相关责任；如引起检疫传染病传播或者有传播严重危

险的，将按照《中华人民共和国刑法》第三百三十二条，处三年以下有期徒刑或者拘役，并处或者单

处罚金。

本人已阅知本申明卡所列事项，保证以上申明内容真实准确。如有虚假申明内容，愿承担相应法律责任。

　　　　　　　　　旅客签名：　　　　　　　　　日期：

　　　　　　　　　　　　　　　　　　　　　　　　　2020 年 3 月 13 日，第五版

健康申明须知

尊敬的旅客朋友，您好！

为有效防范新冠肺炎疫情传播，保护您和他人健康，根据《中华人民共和国国境卫生检疫法》，请您按照中国海关要求，认真、如实填写《健康申明卡》，申报您的健康情况和旅行经历。如您曾在过去14天途经或停留过新冠肺炎疫情高发国家、地区，或目前有发热、乏力、干咳、呼吸困难等症状，请您尽早如实向机组或乘务人员报告。

根据《中华人民共和国刑法》第三百三十二条第一款的有关规定，如有隐瞒或虚假填报，造成疫情传播或有传播严重危险的，将可能被处以三年以下有期徒刑或者拘役等刑事处罚。

您可通过填写纸质版本或通过扫码"海关旅客指尖服务小程序"进行申报。抵达后，请将《健康申明卡》主动提交给海关关员，配合海关做好卫生检疫工作。

感谢您的合作！

EXIT/ENTRY HEALTH DECLARATION FORM OF THE PEOPLE'S REPUBLIC OF CHINA

QR Code for e-Declaration

☐EXIT　☐ENTRY

(Please **tick** one of the boxes with " √ ")

Name:＿＿＿＿＿＿＿＿＿＿＿＿＿＿＿＿＿＿＿＿ Gender: ☐Male　☐Female.

Date of birth:＿＿＿＿＿Year＿＿＿＿＿Month＿＿＿＿＿Day　Occupation:＿＿＿＿＿＿

Nationality (region):＿＿＿＿＿＿＿＿City of residence:＿＿＿＿＿＿＿＿＿＿＿＿

1. Passport No.:＿＿＿＿＿＿Other identity document (please specify) No.:＿＿＿＿＿＿

   Flight (ship/train) No.:＿＿＿＿＿＿＿＿Seat No.:＿＿＿＿＿＿＿＿＿＿＿＿

   Port of exit/entry:＿＿＿＿＿＿＿＿＿Destination:＿＿＿＿＿＿＿＿＿＿＿＿

2. ☐Chinese mobile number and other contact information:＿＿＿＿＿＿＿＿＿＿

   ☐Overseas mobile number and other contact information:＿＿＿＿＿＿＿＿＿

   Contact persons in China and their phone numbers:＿＿＿＿＿＿＿＿＿＿＿＿

   What's your address in the next 14 days? (Please provide detailed address. For address inChina, please specify the street, community, building/house/apartment number, or the address of the hotel)＿＿＿＿＿＿＿＿＿＿＿＿＿＿＿＿＿＿＿＿＿＿＿＿＿＿＿＿＿＿

   If you come (return) to China on (from) a business trip, please specify the inviting person (organization)＿＿＿＿＿＿＿＿and the host person (organization)＿＿＿＿＿＿＿

3. Where have you visited in China during the past 14 days? (Please specify the provinces/autonomous regions/municipalities and cities, including Hong Kong，Macao and Taiwan regions)＿＿＿＿＿＿

   If you have visited other countries and regions during the past 14 days, please specify:＿＿＿＿＿

4. Have you had direct contact with confirmed/suspected/symptomless cases of COVID-19 during the past 14 days? ☐Yes　☐No

   Have you had direct contact with people having fever and/or symptoms of respiratory infection during the past 14 days? ☐Yes　☐No

   Has your community reported any COVID-19 cases during the past 14 days? ☐Yes　☐No

   Have there been two or more members in your office/family having fever and/or symptoms of respiratory infection during the past 14 days? ☐Yes　☐No

5. Do you have now, or have you had in the past 14 days, the following symptoms? ☐Yes　☐No

   If yes, please tick your symptoms with" √ "　☐Fever　☐Chills　☐Dry cough　☐Expectoration ☐Stuffy nose　☐Running nose　☐Sore throat　☐Headache　☐Fatigue　☐Dizziness　☐Muscle pain ☐Arthralgia　☐Shortness of breath　☐Difficulty breathing　☐Chest tightness　☐Chest pain ☐Conjunctival congestion　☐Nausea　☐Vomiting　☐Diarrhea　☐Stomachache　☐Others＿＿＿＿

   ＿＿＿＿＿＿＿＿＿＿＿＿＿＿＿＿＿＿＿＿＿＿＿＿＿＿＿＿＿＿＿＿＿＿

   Have you taken any medications for fever, cold or cough during the past 14 days? ☐Yes　☐No

6. If you have tested for COVID-19 during the past 14 days, is the result positive? ☐Yes　☐No

Dear Passengers, according to relevant laws and regulations, for your health and that of others, please fill out thisExit/Entry Health Declaration Form truthfully. If you conceal or falsely declare the information, you will be held accountable according to the Frontier Health and Quarantine Law of the People's Republic of China, and if the spread of, quarantinable communicable diseases or a serious danger of spreading them is thereby caused, you shall be sentenced to not more than three years of fixed-term imprisonment or criminal detention, and may in addition or exclusively be sentenced to a fine, according to Article 332 of the Criminal Law of the People's Republic of China.

I hereby certify that all the above information is true and correct. I will take the legal responsibility in case of false declaration.

Signature:　　　　　　　　　　　Date:

The fifth edition, published on March 13, 2020

Notice

Dear Passengers,

To effectively contain the spread of COVID-19 and protect your health and that of others, according to the Frontier Health and Quarantine Lawof the People's Republic of China, you are requested to fill out the Exit/Entry Health Declaration Form to declare your health conditions and travel history truthfully. If you have been to, either for a visit or transit,any hard-hit countries or regions during the past 14 days, or if you are showing such symptoms as fever, fatigue, dry cough, difficulty breathing, etc., please report to the crew members immediately.

According to Article 332 of the Criminal Law of the People's Republic of China, anyone who conceals or falsely declares the information, causing the spread of quarantinable communicable diseases or a serious danger of spreading them, shall be sentenced to not more than three years of fixed-term imprisonment, criminal detention or other criminal punishment.

You can complete health declaration either by hand writing or on the WeChat applet. When you arrive, please give your Health Declaration Form to customs officers, and cooperate with them in health quarantine procedures.

Thank you for your cooperation.

参考文献

［1］中国引航协会.关于防控被引船输入性新冠肺炎风险的应对措施：2020-03-06.

China Maritime Pilots' Association. The Prevention and Control Measures for Imported the COVID-19 Infections from Ships under Pilotage: 2020-03-06.

［2］国家卫生健康委办公厅，国家中医药管理局办公室.新型冠状病毒肺炎诊疗方案（试行第七版）：2020-03-04.

General Office of the National Health Commission of the People's Republic of China. COVID-19 Diagnosis and Treatment Plan (Provisional 7th Edition)：2020-03-04.

［3］中华人民共和国海事局.船舶船员新冠肺炎疫情防控操作指南（V1.0）：2020-03-02.

Maritime Safety Administration of the People's Republic of China. Guidance on the prevention and control of COVID-19 on board (Version 1.0): 2020-03-02.

［4］西京医院防控办公室.西京医院新型冠状病毒肺炎防控知识手册.2020-01-30.

［5］截至 3 月 22 日 24 时新型冠状病毒肺炎疫情最新情况．中华人民共和国卫生健康委员会官方网站：2020-03-23.

［6］火神山医院正式交付军方，明日开始收治病人．中华人民共和国卫生健康委员会官方网站：2020-02-03.

［7］湖北将继续采取最严格防控措施．中国日报双语新闻微信公众号：2020-02-25.

［8］严防境外输入 筑牢水上防线．中国交通新闻网：2020-03-10.

［9］全国 346 支医疗队抵达武汉湖北．人民日报微博：2020-03-08.

［10］交通运输部，人力资源和社会保障部．妥善做好疫情期间国际航行船舶在船船员换班安排．中华人民共和国海事局官方网站．2020-03-17.

［11］还敢拒绝隔离、不如实填报健康申明卡？定罪处罚．央广新闻微信公众号：2020-03-16.

［12］五部委再发公告．中国民航网：2020-03-22.

图书在版编目（CIP）数据

船舶驾引人员防控新冠肺炎英语手册：英汉对照/中国航海学会，中国引航协会，杨炳栋编.—上海：上海浦江教育出版社有限公司，2020.5

ISBN 978-7-81121-649-3

Ⅰ.①船… Ⅱ.①中… ②中… ③杨… Ⅲ.①日冕形病毒—病毒病—肺炎—预防（卫生）—手册—英、汉 Ⅳ.①R563.101-62

中国版本图书馆CIP数据核字（2020）第069023号

上海浦江教育出版社出版发行

社址：上海海港大道1550号上海海事大学校内　　邮政编码：201306

电话：（021）38284912（发行）　　38284923（总编室）　　38284910（传真）

E-mail: cbs@shmtu.edu.cn　URL: http://www.pujiangpress.cn

上海商务联西印刷有限公司印装

幅面尺寸：125 mm × 185 mm　　印张：4.25　　字数：92千字

2020年5月第1版　　2020年5月第1次印刷

责任编辑：张怡　杨川

定价：15.00元